Pescatarian Cookbook for Beginners

The Complete Meal Prep Guide for Healthy Eating and Weight Loss with Easy Fish and Seafood Recipes and Weekly Meal Plans

Stella Allen

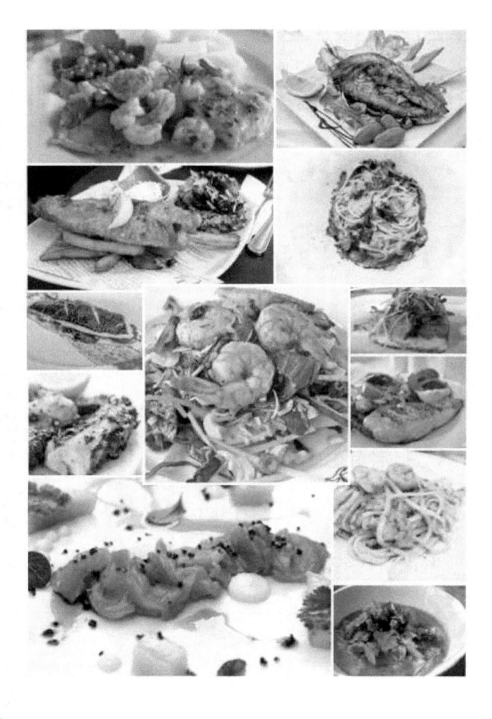

Text Copyright©

Legal & Disclaimer

Upon using the contents and information contained in this book, you agree to hold harmless the Author from and against any damages, costs, and expenses, including any legal fees potentially resulting from the application of any of the information provided by this book. This disclaimer applies to any loss, damages or injury caused by the use and application, whether directly or indirectly, of any advice or information presented, whether for breach of contract, tort, negligence, personal injury, criminal intent, or under any other cause of action.

You agree to accept all risks of using the information presented inside this book.

You agree that by continuing to read this book, where appropriate and/or necessary, you shall consult a professional (including but not limited to your doctor, attorney, or financial advisor or such needed) before using any of the suggested remedies, techniques, or information in this book.

Table of Contents

Introduction

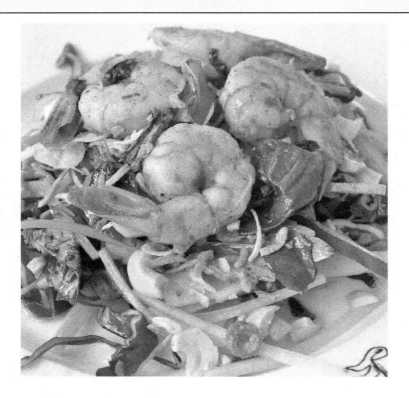

The term pescatarian derives from the combination of the words "pesce" and "vegetarian". "Pesce" comes from the Italian language, meaning fish. This diet is seen as part of the vegetarian spectrum because it contains a large amount of plant-based foods. A pescatarian does not eat meat, but they do eat fish and seafood.

People often choose a pescatarian diet for health reasons, environmental concerns, and/or ethical reasons.

A pescatarian diet lowers the risk of having chronic medical problems, such as heart disease. Seafood generally has a lower amount of fat and cholesterol than most meats, which is beneficial to the health of your heart. Fatty fish contain omega-3 fatty acids (DHA and EPA), which also promote a healthy heart. DHA and EPA are linked to a decrease in high blood pressure and decrease the risk of heart disease. They may also lesson symptoms of rheumatoid arthritis and can be preventative of heart attacks. Stricter diets such as the vegetarian and vegan diet increase your risk of having a vitamin or mineral deficiency, as well as having fewer options for protein sources. Pescatarians can easily source these much-needed vitamins and minerals by eating a wide variety of seafood, whole grains and produce.

Fish contain many nutrients and minerals such as vitamin D, B2 (riboflavin), iron, zinc, iodine, magnesium, potassium and more. Fish is also rich in calcium and phosphorus, which are beneficial for bone health. Zinc is especially present in oysters, while mussels are a great source for iron and selenium. Clams are also rich in selenium, as well as calcium.

There are many environmental concerns regarding meat eating diets. Meat production creates greenhouse gases and harms the environment. There are higher amounts of carbon emissions, increased land use, and an increase use of resources. Livestock release a substantial amount of methane, a greenhouse gas much more potent than carbon dioxide. The feed production that is used to fatten the livestock requires large amounts of fertilizer, fuel, pesticides and water. This takes millions of acres of cropland as well as millions of pounds of pesticides and fertilizer. The manure of the livestock, as well as the processing of the livestock and transportation of animals yields a great amount of pollution and waste. These are just a few of the environmental concerns regarding meat consumption, and a pescatarian diet will allow you to decrease the impact you have on the environment.

Many of the ethical reasons that people choose to pursue a pescatarian diet have to do with environmental concerns, as well as the treatment of animals. Some people also disagree with poor labor conditions and pursue this diet for humanitarian reasons.

Some of these reasons include: not wanting to partake in killing animals for food, disagreeing with inhumane factory practices, not wanting to support the poor labor conditions that workers experience, and disagreeing with the land and resource use for animal feed and production because it is unjust.

If you are seeking a well-rounded healthy diet, wanting to decrease your environmental footprint, or agree with any of the ethical reasons, a pescatarian diet may be the ideal route for you.

The Pescatarian Diet

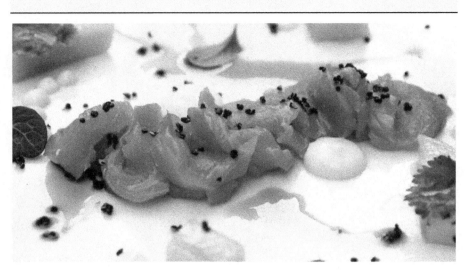

Seafood-Based

While seafood can certainly be a decadent treat for special occasions, there are also many benefits in consuming it on a regular basis. Here are a few of them:

- Eating more fish and seafood regularly can reduce the risk of obesity. Both fish and seafood are low in calories and saturated fat but high in protein and healthy fats, which means they will keep you fuller longer. If you're being calorie conscious, get your daily intake by eating more fish without going overboard on butter or oil.

- The American Heart Association recommends all healthy adults consume fish at least twice a week to prevent cardiovascular diseases such as stroke. The high levels of HDL (the "good" cholesterol) in fish can help lower overall cholesterol levels.

- Fish is a brain booster! Researchers from the Ronald Reagan UCLA Medical Center have found that consumption of baked or broiled fish on a regular basis is linked to higher functionality in areas of the brain that are responsible for comprehension and recollection in adults. Eating fish can also prevent plaque buildup in the brain, which is believed to be one of the causes of Alzheimer's disease.

- Consuming fish can have a significant impact on mental health. Fatty fish such as salmon contains high levels of protein, selenium, and omega-3s, which can help balance mood and lower the risk of depression.

A common concern people have with seafood and fish is the potential for high levels of mercury. Mercury is toxic to a child's developing brain and nervous system, so the Food and Drug Administration warns women who may become pregnant, are pregnant, or are nursing to avoid fish with high amounts of mercury. A general rule of thumb is that the larger (and more predatory) the fish, the higher the mercury, and since mercury is present in fish, the concentrations increase the more a fish eats other fish.

According to the National Resources Defense Council, some fish and seafood that are low in mercury are catfish, clams, crab, salmon, sardines, shrimp, tilapia, and freshwater trout. Some fish that contain higher levels of mercury are grouper, king mackerel, swordfish, orange roughy, and bigeye and ahi tuna. As with most things, eating fish high in mercury is generally okay as long as it is consumed sparingly.

TIPS TO ELIMINATE FISHY SMELL

Fresh fish shouldn't have a very strong odor. It should smell like the sea water (or lake water) from which it was caught. If the fish is really fresh, it should give off a briny ocean smell. Sometimes, though, that "fishy" odor can turn you off from eating it.

So, what's with that fishy smell? According to the American Society for Nutrition, the smell associated with fish comes from their physiology. Fish use certain amino acids to help balance salt levels in their cells. When the fish are killed, bacteria and enzymes convert the amino acids to another compound that gives off that fishy odor.

You can reduce the odor in a few ways:

1. Make sure the fish is fresh. Rinse the fish with cold water to wash away any surface compounds and treat the fish with an acidic ingredient such as lemon, vinegar, or tomato. Acid makes the bacteria and enzymes bind with water instead of with more of the amino acids, decreasing the odor.

2. Discard the packaging and empty the garbage immediately after prepping the fish. This will keep the odor from spreading throughout your house.

3. Use the range hood or open a window to circulate fresh air.

4. After rinsing the fish, scrub your sink clean and sprinkle baking soda or sliced lemons down your garbage disposal. Again, acidic environments can prevent the odor-causing compounds from doing their thing.

Plant-Based Meals

It is essential to mention that consuming healthy plant-based meals is not the only thing that will provide you with a healthy life. Also, it is crucial to work out regularly; live a stress-free life, quit smoking and drinking, and is psychologically in a good place.

This is what we know from the medical researches so far:

Heart Disease

Vegetarians have a lower risk for cardiac diseases (mainly heart attack) and death from heart failures.

In a study published a few years ago, that involved more than seventy thousand participants, on average the vegetarians had a 25% lower risk of dying from heart failures

In another study with more than sixty thousand participants (mainly people in the Oxford cohort of the European Prospective Investigation into Cancer and Nutrition (EPIC-Oxford)), the vegetarians had a 19% lower risk of death from heart issues.

If you want to keep your heart in good health, the best thing is to eat whole-grain foods and legumes (high in fiber). Such foods keep the blood sugar levels in balance and reduce the levels of cholesterol.

Nuts are an excellent food for the heart. They contain a low glycemic index and multiple antioxidants, fiber, vegetable protein, minerals, and good fatty acids. On the other hand, nuts are packed in calories and should be consumed in small amounts. But the great thing is that even a small amount will keep you full.

For example, walnuts are rich in omega-3 fatty acids, known for their numerous health benefits.

Fish is the best source of omega-3 fatty acids (which in some of the vegetarian types of diet is allowed). But, plant-derived omega-3 fatty acids may not be the ideal substitute for fish.

Cancer

Regularly eating fruits and vegetables will lower the risk of developing malignant diseases such as cancer. There is no scientific evidence that the vegetarian diet will protect you from this illness. Still, hundreds of studies show that the vegetarian diet will provide you with the daily needed servings of vegetables and fruits.

You can give up on meat for a while (no matter if you want to become a vegetarian or not), and you will reduce the risk of colon cancer. Vegetarians are known to have a lower risk of consuming foods that will remain cancer genic substances in their colons.

Type 2 diabetes

Plant-based diets are known to reduce the risk of type 2 diabetes. Vegetarians are not as exposed to the risk of this illness as non-vegetarians are.

According to the Harvard-based Women's Health Study, there is a link between eating red meat (mainly processed meats – hot dogs, bacon, and salami) and diabetes risk.

Bone health

As women age, their bone health tends to get weaker. Osteoporosis is widespread (bones are exposed to a higher risk of fractures). This is why some women are not prone to switching to the vegetarian diet. The reason for that is that the vegetarian diet is reducing the number of dairy products, which are the primary source for healthy bones.

If the health of your bones is your priority, you can always pick one of the types of vegetarian diets, such as lacto-ovo vegetarians (where you are allowed to consume dairy products and eggs). This type of vegetarian diet provides you with enough calcium (almost as much as a regular meat-eater gets on a daily basis).

Besides dairy products and eggs, some vegetables like broccoli, bok choy, Chinese cabbage, kale, and collards are rich in calcium. Also, Swiss chard and spinach contain calcium, but they are not the best choices because, besides calcium, they contain oxalates that make it harder for your body to absorb the calcium.

Fruits and vegetables that are rich in potassium and magnesium are excellent for reducing the blood acidity, which will lower the risk of the elimination of calcium through the urine.

Vegetarians (particularly vegans) are at higher risk of not getting enough amounts of vitamins K and D that are needed for bone health. Some leafy greens do contain vitamin K. If your choice is veganism, you should include leafy greens in your diet, as well as organic orange juice, rice, and soy milk and cereals, as well as taking the vitamin D supplement.

How to Prepare Your Pescatarian Kitchen

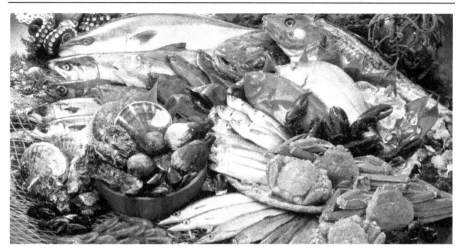

As a dietitian, one of my favorite catchphrases is "Proper planning provides for peak performance!" While it may be hard to say that five times fast, it couldn't be truer than when developing healthy eating habits, like adopting the pescatarian diet.

Without preparation, it's easy to make excuses. Think about it—how many times have you said something like "I don't have beans [or insert any pantry item], so I can't make the bean tacos [or any recipe] I planned. I'll just order takeout instead." One missed dinner turns into two, which turns into several. You forget to restock your pantry, and over time you begin to feel the effects of too much takeout. You're lethargic, bloated from excess salt, and even pack on a few unwanted pounds.

Instead, be prepared for success on the pescatarian diet: stock your pantry, take inventory, and get organized. This way, you'll feel confident in what you're doing. Having a well-stocked kitchen and pantry helps eliminate common obstacles and improves your organization. Frequently used ingredients will be available, you'll cut trips to the supermarket in half, and you'll save time and money. Even more, studies show that being organized can help improve your healthy eating habits and boost your energy, so let's get started.

STOCKING THE ESSENTIALS

Setting a good foundation in your kitchen will help spur your success in adopting the pescatarian lifestyle. First, get prepared. Second, take inventory of your current pantry, refrigerator, and freezer. You may have more than you think! Surveying your inventory will help you save money by avoiding duplicate purchases. This is also a good time to toss expired pantry items (or those with too much freezer burn). Organize your pantry using the "first in, first out" system to prevent waste in the future. Place items with a sooner expiration date closer to the front and those with a later date behind them. Next, eliminate what you don't need or use. Donate these items to a local food pantry. Finally, stock up to save time later. Head to the store to restock your pantry, refrigerator, and freezer with the necessities to succeed on a pescatarian plan.

The Pantry

Canned beans: Canned beans are one of the most flexible and inexpensive plant-based proteins to stock in your pantry. Full of fiber, too, canned beans can be used in salads, soups, snacks, main dishes, and even desserts (you must try the Blender Black Bean Brownies).

Canned salmon: As an inexpensive alternative to fresh-caught salmon, canned salmon is packed with protein, omega-3 fatty acids, and even calcium (if it contains bones). For a fraction of the price, you can always eat the pescatarian way if you have canned salmon (and other fish, like sardines and tuna) in your pantry.

Chia seeds: These tiny black seeds are a nutritious superstar and versatile in the kitchen. Sprinkle them on any dish for an extra nutritious boost as they contain a balance of healthy fats, plant-based protein, and fiber. Plus, when added to liquid, chia seeds gel, absorbing up to nine times their weight in liquid and creating a pudding-like texture.

Diced canned tomatoes: Did you know that US-grown canned tomatoes go from farm to can within hours? This locks in their nutrients, including lycopene, vitamins C and E, and potassium, so you get the most out of this seasonal fruit. Plus, canned tomatoes contain more of the antioxidant lycopene than fresh tomatoes, which helps reduce inflammation and ward off chronic diseases.

Dry whole-grains (farro, buckwheat, bulgur, quinoa, etc.): Whole-grains are a staple on the pescatarian diet because they're high in fiber, vitamins, and minerals. Replacing refined white grains with whole-grains will boost your heart health, improve blood sugar control, and more. There are more than 20 types of whole-grains to choose from, so have fun experimenting over time.

Quality oils: Not all oils are created equally. opt for pure heart-healthy oils rich in monounsaturated fats, like olive oil and avocado oil. Avocado oil is the preferred option for higher cooking temperatures because of its higher smoke point, while olive oil is used in dressings and marinades; however, both can safely be used interchangeably.

Rolled oats: A deliciously nutritious breakfast staple, multipurpose oats are rich in fiber, B vitamins, magnesium, iron, and more, plus they're inexpensive.

Spices: A well-stocked spice rack is one of the easiest ways to enhance the flavor of your meal without adding fat or calories. Many spices contain unique health benefits from warding off the common cold to easing digestive discomfort. If you're just building your spice cabinet, start with the basics salt, pepper, garlic powder, oregano, cinnamon, red pepper flakes, smoked paprika, cumin, chili powder, and curry powder.

The Refrigerator

Avocados: Rich in healthy fats, fiber, and antioxidants, avocados are a "superfood" you should have on hand to mash on toast, add to smoothies, turn into sauces and dressings, throw in a salad, or use in burgers like the Tuna Avocado Burgers. When shopping finds, avocados that are soft to squeeze, but not mushy. If you remove the stem at the top, it should be green, not brown.

Eggs: Eggs are a quick, easy, and versatile protein source to stock in your refrigerator. When possible, look for the terms "organic," "free-range," and "no added hormones." Although "pasture-raised" is not a regulated term, these eggs have been found to contain more anti-inflammatory omega-3 fatty acids and vitamin D.

Fresh fish and shellfish: You'll learn how to select the best fish, but always ask your fishmonger what's freshest when at the fish counter.

Fresh herbs: Add fresh herbs for a bright burst of flavor and plenty of health benefits, too. Parsley, cilantro, dill, rosemary, and thyme are just a few favorites featured throughout the recipes in this book.

Fruit: Most Americans do not consume the recommended two to three servings of fruit per day. Stock your refrigerator with your favorites so you always have an easy snack option. Berries, apples, and pears contain the most fiber, but also shop for melons, bananas, and stone fruits for variety.

Organic tofu: Tofu is an excellent source of plant-based protein and calcium, which is why it's perfect for the pescatarian diet. Organic tofu is inexpensive and GMO-free.

Vegetables: You can't go wrong when stocking your refrigerator with vegetables. When shopping, your cart should look like a rainbow.

The Freezer

Frozen fish: Frozen fish is an affordable way to incorporate seafood into your diet. Minimal nutrients, if any, are lost in the freezing process.

Frozen fruit: Frozen fruit is typically more affordable than fresh, and it's a great option for off-season fruit. It's picked and frozen at its peak ripeness, which also means its peak nutrient content.

Frozen vegetables: If you often let fresh vegetables spoil, opt for frozen! Picked, processed, and frozen at their peak ripeness, frozen vegetables are an excellent alternative to fresh.

The Hardware

You don't need a Michelin-star-worthy kitchen to follow the pescatarian diet. Aside from an oven and stove, plus basic kitchen utensils (like a spatula, ladle, and tongs), here are five kitchen essentials that will help you eat the pescatarian way:

Nesting mixing bowls: Whether you're making a salad, mixing cookie dough, or prepping vegetables to roast, a set of nesting mixing bowls will be helpful in your kitchen. If possible, find a set with matching lids for easy storage in your refrigerator.

Parchment paper: For easy cleanup, parchment paper is a must-have in your pescatarian kitchen. Line sheet pans with parchment paper when roasting vegetables or baking fish to reduce cleaning time. Preparing fish en papillote, or in a pouch made from parchment paper, is a simple and quick technique, too.

Sauté pan or cast-iron pan: The best way to get crispy skin on fish is to pan-sear it on your stovetop. A heavy sauté pan or cast-iron pan is the best kitchen tool to use for this. Bonus points if your pan is oven safe!

Sharp chef's knife: Investing in a good chef's knife, and knowing how to use it, will make prep time a breeze! Alongside a good knife, having a sturdy cutting board that doesn't slide with each cut is important.

Sheet pans: Whether you're roasting, baking, or broiling, sheet pans are necessary to get the job done. Look for rimmed sheet pans to prevent spills in your oven.

SMART SPENDING

The pescatarian diet can cost a pretty penny since seafood is one of the most expensive proteins available. You can be a smart shopper and spend less, however, by following these tips:

1. Plan your meals to avoid waste.

2. Choose frozen over fresh. Frozen seafood, vegetables, fruit, and even grains can be more affordable than their fresh counterparts. In fact, much of the fish you see "fresh" at the fish counter was previously frozen (check the signs and ask your fishmonger). Even more, you don't have to worry about waste as much when buying frozen foods, since they last longer and don't have to be used right away.

3. Eat seasonally. In-season produce and fish are less expensive, so plan your meals accordingly. For example, in many parts of the country crab season is in the fall and winter. Reserve your crab intake for these months to get the biggest bang for your buck!

4. Use a bulk frozen fish delivery service. There are several frozen food delivery services that allow you to purchase high-quality fish and shellfish in bulk at discounted prices. Frozen is just as nutritious as fresh, so don't be shy about using these services (if you have the freezer space).

5. Shop for staples online. Oftentimes, buying nonperishable staples, including dry grains, canned beans, canned tomatoes, canned fish, and oil online can save you money. Just as you may

price-compare your local supermarkets, shop around online between different vendors to find the best deals.

SELECTING AND PREPARING FISH AND SEAFOOD

Is preparing fish and shellfish intimidating to you? You're not alone. Maybe it's the scaly skin, hard shells, or googly eyes staring back at you. Perhaps it's fear of a fishy scent lingering throughout your home. Or maybe previous attempts resulted in a dry, overpriced home experiment that didn't turn out favorably. Whatever fishy beliefs you may have, purchasing, preparing, and cooking seafood is much easier than you think.

In fact, you don't have to worry about many of these common obstacles if you're just getting started. There are foolproof ways to master cooking fish at home.

What and What Not to Eat

What do Pescatarians Eat?

- Peanuts and seeds, nuts and nut butter
- Whole grains and grain products
- Vegetables
- Fruits
- Seeds including flaxseeds, chia, and hemp
- Legumes including lentils, hummus, tofu and beans
- Dairy including cheese, milk, and yogurt
- Shellfish and fish

- Eggs

What not to Eat

- Pork

- Turkey

- Chicken

- Beef

- Lamb

- Wild game

Essential Pescatarian Food Preparation Tips

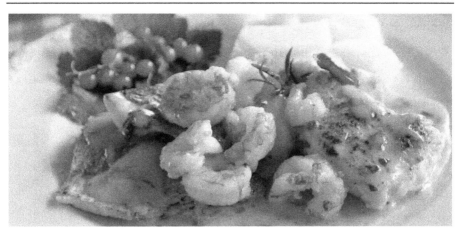

Before delving deep into preparing Pescatarian cuisine, here are some practical tips to help make your cooking experiences more rewarding and tasteful.

Seafood handling and safety

Seafood can be tricky. Its shelf life without refrigeration is typically shorter than meats and poultry. Also, it does not hold up well as a leftover, unless it is fried with thick coats of breadcrumbs. Cooked seafood is not as appetizing as roast beef or baked chicken after a week in the refrigerator.

Contamination can also be a problem. Fish breathe air in a different environment than other sources of protein. These environments can be contaminated and fishermen may be unaware of chemicals introduced into their environment. Though it might be a little more expensive, seafood should be bought from reputable outlets. It is also a good idea to find out what area they come from. Seafood should be cleaned and washed thoroughly before preparation in order to minimize contamination.

Unless seafood is consumed in a restaurant, preparation of raw seafood recipes, such as sashimi and sushi, should be left in the hands of capable restaurant personnel. Seafood must be well (not over) cooked for safe consumption.

Ingredients

In keeping with the healthy theme of the Pescetarian diet, recipe ingredients should have the least possible amounts of saturated fat, refined sugars, preservatives, and chemical additives. Virgin olive oil and coconut oil should be used instead of other cooking oils containing high levels of unsaturated or "trans fats" present in most vegetable oils. When adding eggs to a dish, try to stay with eggs from naturally fed hens, or eggs that are infused with Omega-3 oils. Refined sugar should be substituted with natural sweeteners, if possible. Instead of refined table salt, consider using coarse sea salt or sodium reduced salt.

As for condiments, it is always a good choice to go natural, especially for the spices, such as basil, coriander, and dill weed. The alternatives are powdered and/or dried herbs that can be used without sacrificing much of the intended flavor.

Preparation Methods

There will be few recipes here that will involve a little sautéing, but try to avoid frying if at all possible. While frying may appear to be the easiest and safest way to cook seafood, it actually sends most of the nutrients to the un-consumed pool of oil at the bottom of the pan.

Frying also increases the fat content of the dish. When fish is deep-fried in high temperatures, there is also a risk of forming toxic by-products. There are many alternatives for preparing delicious seafood, including baking, poaching, broiling, grilling, and pan roasting. Also, remember that the recommended internal cooking temperature of fish is around 145 degrees.

Benefits of Adding Fish to a Vegetarian Diet

You will enjoy several benefits when you add fish to the vegetarian diet. Several people are worried that avoiding animal flesh or totally eliminating animal products could cause a low intake of certain vital nutrients. For instance, it is tough to get protein, calcium, zinc, and vitamin B12 on a vegan diet. When you add seafood like mollusks, crustaceans, and fish to the vegetarian diet, you will begin to enjoy vital nutrients and varieties in your diet.

- Get more omega-3s

The best way to get omega-3 fatty acids is by consuming fish. Some plant-based foods like flaxseed walnuts contain alpha-linolenic acid, which is a type of omega-3 fat. But it is not easy for the body to convert this type of acid to docosahexaenoic acid DHA and eicosapentaenoic acid (EPA). EPA and DHA have more benefits that are helpful to the heart, brain, and mood. Oily fish like sardines and salmon contain both DHA and EPA.

- Boost your protein intake

Every person needs a daily intake of about 0.8g of protein per 2.2 pounds of body weight to stay healthy. So, a person who weighs 150 pounds needs to eat a minimum of 54 grams of protein daily. It can be tough to achieve a high protein diet with just plant-based foods, particularly if you do not want extra fat or carbs with your protein. An excellent source of lean protein is fish and other seafood, as it gives your body the protein needed for the body to perform optimally.

- Seafood has other nutrients

Apart from protein and omega-3s, seafood is rich in several other nutrients. For example, oysters have a high content of vitamin B12, selenium, and zinc. One oyster gives 55 percent of the RDI for selenium and zinc, as well as 133 percent of the RDI for vitamin B12.

Mussel is another seafood that has high contents of selenium, manganese, vitamin B12, and other B vitamins.

White fish varieties like flounder and cod do not have much omega-3 fats but provide extremely lean protein. For instance, 3 ounces of cod produces less than a gram of fat and 19 grams of protein. Cod is a great choice for people who need niacin, phosphorus, selenium, vitamins B6 and vitamins B12

Substitutions and More Tips to Remember

While the recipes here specify certain fish types, you can substitute some fish types for those specified. Certain fish types, such as salmon, tuna, and Chilean sea bass, have more fat content than other varieties (typically about 5%). As a result, these types are more flavorful than "lean" fish, such as tilapia, cod or halibut. Once again, remember that more fish fat, to an extent, is good for you because of the Omega-3 oils.

Of course, the leaner fish types have their own strengths. They tend to have a firmer consistency and texture, which makes them the perfect choice for stews, chowders, and soups.

Most fishes can be used interchangeably. However, it is a good idea to talk to your grocer if you plan to substitute seafood types before you cook.

Now, let's cook!

Pescatarian Breakfast

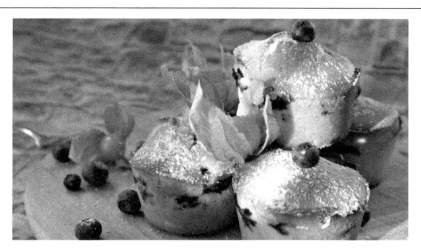

1. Whole-Wheat Blueberry Muffins

Preparation Time: 5 Minutes

Cooking Time: 25 Minutes

Servings: 8

Ingredients:

- ½ cup plant-based milk (here or here)
- ½ cup unsweetened applesauce
- ½ cup maple syrup
- 1 teaspoon vanilla extract
- 2 cups whole-wheat flour
- ½ teaspoon baking soda
- 1 cup blueberries

Directions:

1. Preheat the oven to 375°F.

2. In a large bowl, mix together the milk, applesauce, maple syrup, and vanilla.

3. Stir in the flour and baking soda until no dry flour is left and the batter is smooth.

4. Gently fold in the blueberries until they are evenly distributed throughout the batter.

5. In a muffin tin, fill 8 muffin cups three-quarters full of batter.

6. Bake for 25 minutes, or until you can stick a knife into the center of a muffin and it comes out clean. Allow to cool before serving.

Nutrition: Calories: 200 Total fat: 1g Carbohydrates: 45g Fiber: 2g Protein: 4g

2. Walnut Crunch Banana Bread

Preparation time: 5 minutes

Cooking time: 1 Hour, plus 30 Minutes to Cool

Servings: 5

Ingredients:

- 4 ripe bananas
- ¼ cup maple syrup
- 1 tablespoon apple cider vinegar
- 1 teaspoon vanilla extract
- 1½ cups whole-wheat flour
- ½ teaspoon ground cinnamon
- ½ teaspoon baking soda
- ¼ cup walnut pieces (optional)

Directions:

1. Preheat the oven to 350°F.
2. In a large bowl, use a fork or mixing spoon to mash the bananas until they reach a puréed consistency (small bits of banana are fine). Stir in the maple syrup, apple cider vinegar, and vanilla.
3. Stir in the flour, cinnamon, and baking soda. Fold in the walnut pieces (if using).
4. Gently pour the batter into a loaf pan, filling it no more than three-quarters of the way full. Bake for 1 hour, or until you can stick a knife into the middle and it comes out clean.
5. Remove from the oven and allow cooling on the countertop for a minimum of 30 minutes before serving.

Nutrition: Calories: 178 Total fat: 1g Carbohydrates: 40g Fiber: 5g Protein: 4g

3. Plant-Powered Pancakes

Preparation time: 5 minutes

Cooking time: 15 minutes

Servings: 8

Ingredients:

- 1 cup whole-wheat flour
- 1 teaspoon baking powder
- ½ teaspoon ground cinnamon
- 1 cup plant-based milk (here or here)
- ½ cup unsweetened applesauce
- ¼ cup maple syrup
- 1 teaspoon vanilla extract

Directions:

1. In a large bowl, combine the flour, baking powder, and cinnamon.
2. Stir in the milk, applesauce, maple syrup, and vanilla until no dry flour is left and the batter is smooth.
3. Heat a large, nonstick skillet or griddle over medium heat. For each pancake, pour ¼ cup of batter onto the hot skillet. Once bubbles form over the top of the pancake and the sides begin to brown, flip and cook for 1 to 2 minutes more.
4. Repeat until all of the batter is used, and serve.

Nutrition: Calories: 210 Total fat: 2g Carbohydrates: 44g Fiber: 5g Protein: 5g

4. Maple-Pecan Granola

Preparation time: 5 minutes

Cooking time: 20 minutes

Servings: 4

Ingredients:

- 1½ cups rolled oats
- ¼ cup pecan pieces
- ¼ cup maple syrup
- 1 teaspoon vanilla extract
- ½ teaspoon ground cinnamon

Directions:

1. Preheat the oven to 300°F. Line a baking sheet with parchment paper.
2. In a large bowl, combine the oats, pecan pieces, maple syrup, vanilla, and cinnamon. Stir until the oats and pecan pieces are completely coated.
3. Spread the mixture on the baking sheet in an even layer. Bake for 20 minutes, stirring once after 10 minutes.
4. Remove from the oven, and allow cooling on the countertop for 30 minutes before serving. The granola may still be a bit soft right after you remove it from the oven, but it will gradually firm up as it cools.

Nutrition: Calories: 220 Total fat: 7g Carbohydrates: 35g Fiber: 4g Protein: 5g

5. Paradise Island Overnight Oatmeal

Preparation time: 5 minutes

Cooking time: 0 minutes

Servings: 2

Ingredients:

- 2 cups rolled oats
- 2 cups plant-based milk (here or here)
- ½ cup diced mango (fresh or frozen)
- ½ cup pineapple chunks (fresh or frozen)
- 1 banana, sliced
- 1 tablespoon maple syrup
- 1 tablespoon chia seeds

Directions:

1. In a large bowl, mix together the oats, milk, mango, pineapple, banana, maple syrup, and chia seeds.
2. Cover and refrigerate overnight or for a minimum of 4 hours before serving.

Nutrition: Calories: 510 Total fat: 12g Carbohydrates: 93g Fiber: 15g Protein: 14g

6. Pumpkin Pie Oatmeal

Preparation time: 5 minutes

Cooking time: 35 minutes

Servings: 4

Ingredients:

- 3 cups plant-based milk (here or here)
- 1 cup steel-cut oats
- 1 cup unsweetened pumpkin purée
- 2 tablespoons maple syrup
- 1 teaspoon ground cinnamon
- ⅛ Teaspoon ground cloves
- ⅛ Teaspoon ground nutmeg

Directions:

1. In a medium saucepan over medium-high heat, bring the milk to a boil. When a rolling boil is reached, reduce the heat to low, and stir in the oats, pumpkin purée, maple syrup, cinnamon, cloves, and nutmeg.
2. Cover and cook for 30 minutes, stirring every few minutes to ensure none of the oatmeal sticks to the bottom of the pot, and serve.

Nutrition: Calories: 218 Total fat: 5g Carbohydrates: 38g Fiber: 6g Protein: 7g

7. Chocolate and Peanut Butter Quinoa

Preparation time: 5 minutes

Cooking time: 10 minutes

Servings: 2

Ingredients:

- 1 cup plant-based milk (here or here)
- 2 cups cooked quinoa (see here)
- 1 tablespoon maple syrup
- 1 tablespoon cocoa powder
- 1 tablespoon defatted peanut powder

Directions:

1. In a medium saucepan over medium-high heat, bring the milk to a boil.
2. Once a rolling boil is reached, reduce the heat to low, and stir in the quinoa, maple syrup, cocoa powder, and peanut powder.
3. Cook, uncovered, for 5 minutes, stirring every other minute. Serve warm.

Nutrition: Calories: 339 Total fat: 8g Carbohydrates: 53g Fiber: 7g Protein: 14g

8. A.M. Breakfast Scramble

Preparation time: 5 minutes

Cooking time: 5 minutes

Servings: 2

Ingredients:
- 1 (14-ounce) package firm or extra-firm tofu
- 4 ounces mushrooms, sliced
- ½ bell pepper, diced
- 2 tablespoons nutritional yeast
- 1 tablespoon vegetable broth or water
- ½ teaspoon garlic powder
- ½ teaspoon onion powder
- ⅛ Teaspoon freshly ground black pepper
- 1 cup fresh spinach

Directions:
1. Heat a large skillet over medium-low heat.
2. Drain the tofu, then place it in the skillet and mash it down with a fork or mixing spoon. Stir in the mushrooms, bell pepper, nutritional yeast, broth, garlic powder, onion powder, and pepper. Cover and cook for 10 minutes, stirring once after about 5 minutes.
3. Uncover, and stir in the spinach. Cook for an additional 5 minutes before serving.

Nutrition: Calories: 230 Total fat: 10g Carbohydrates: 16g Fiber: 7g Protein: 27g

9. Loaded Breakfast Burrito

Preparation time: 5 minutes

Cooking time: 20 minutes

Servings: 2

Ingredients:

- ½ block (7 ounces) firm tofu
- 2 medium potatoes cut into ¼-inch dice
- 1 cup cooked black beans (see here), drained and rinsed
- 4 ounces mushrooms, sliced
- 1 jalapeño, seeded and diced
- 2 tablespoons vegetable broth or water
- 1 tablespoon nutritional yeast
- ½ teaspoon garlic powder
- ½ teaspoon onion powder
- ¼ cup salsa
- 6 corn tortillas

Directions:

1. Heat a large skillet over medium-low heat.
2. Drain the tofu, then place it in the pan and mash it down with a fork or mixing spoon.
3. Stir the potatoes, black beans, mushrooms, jalapeño, broth, nutritional yeast, garlic powder, and onion powder into the skillet. Reduce the heat to low, cover, and cook for 10 minutes, or until the potatoes can be easily pierced with a fork.

4. Uncover, and stir in the salsa. Cook for 5 minutes, stirring every other minute.

5. Warm the tortillas in a microwave for 15 to 30 seconds or in a warm oven until soft.

6. Remove the pan from the heat, place one-sixth of the filling in the center of each tortilla, and roll the tortillas into burritos before serving.

Nutrition: Calories: 535 Total fat: 8g Carbohydrates: 95g Fiber: 21g Protein: 29g

Pescatarian Main Meals

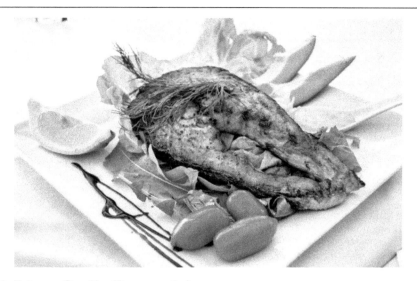

10. Lime Garlic Roasted Asparagus

Preparation time: 5 minutes

Cooking time: 10 minutes

Servings: 2

Ingredients:

- 8 ounces asparagus

- ½ teaspoon minced garlic

- ¼ of lime, zested, sliced

- 1 tablespoon olive oil

- 2 tablespoons grated parmesan cheese

Extra:

- 1/3 teaspoon salt

- ¼ teaspoon ground black pepper

- 1/8 teaspoon dried thyme

- ¼ teaspoon onion powder

Directions:

1. Switch on the oven, then set it to 425 degrees F and let it preheat.

2. Meanwhile, take a medium baking sheet, line it with parchment sheet, and then spread evenly on it.

3. Drizzle asparagus with ½ tablespoon oil and then sprinkle with lime zest, salt, black pepper, thyme, and onion powder.

4. Top asparagus with lime slices and then bake for 5 minutes, tossing halfway.

5. Then stir together garlic and remaining oil, drizzle this mixture over asparagus, toss until mixed, and then continue baking for 2 minutes.

6. When done, sprinkle cheese on top of asparagus and then serve.

7. Meal Prep Instructions:

8. Cool the roasted asparagus and then divide evenly between two meal prep containers. Sprinkle cheese over asparagus, cover with a lid and then store the containers in the refrigerator for up to 5 days. When ready to eat, reheat in the microwave oven for 1 to 2 minutes until hot and then serve.

Nutrition: 115 Cal; 8.5 g Fats; 3.3 g Protein; 5.3 g Carb; 2.6 g Fiber

11. Eggplant Stacks

Preparation time: 5 minutes

Cooking time: 10 minutes

Servings: 2

Ingredients:
- ½ pound, eggplant
- ½ teaspoon dried thyme
- ½ teaspoon dried oregano
- 2 tablespoons olive oil
- 4 tablespoons grated parmesan cheese

Extra:
- ½ teaspoon salt
- ½ teaspoon ground black pepper

Directions:
1. Cut eggplant into 1-inch thick slices, brush them with oil and then sprinkle with salt, black pepper, thyme, and oregano on both until well-seasoned.
2. Take a grill pan, place it over medium heat, grease it with oil and when hot, place seasoned eggplant slices on it, and then grill for 3 to 4 minutes per side until tender.
3. Then top eggplant slices with cheese, cover with a lid, and grill for 1 to 2 minutes until cheese has melted.
4. Serve straight away.
5. Meal Prep Instructions:
6. Cool the eggplant slices, divide them evenly between two meal prep containers, and then store the containers in the refrigerator for up to 5 days. When ready to eat, reheat in the microwave oven for 1 to 2 minutes until hot and then serve.

Nutrition: 200 Cal; 17 g Fats; 4.5 g Protein; 7.5 g Carb; 3.4 g Fiber;

12. Teriyaki Eggplant

Preparation time: 5 minutes

Cooking time: 15 minutes

Servings: 2

Ingredients:

- ½ pound eggplant
- 1 green onion, chopped
- ½ teaspoon grated ginger
- ½ teaspoon minced garlic
- 1/3 cup soy sauce

Extra:

- 1 tablespoon coconut sugar
- ½ tablespoon apple cider vinegar
- 1 tablespoon olive oil

Directions:

1. Prepare teriyaki sauce and for this, take a medium bowl, add ginger, garlic, soy sauce, vinegar, and sugar in it and then whisk until sugar has dissolved completely.

2. Cut eggplant into cubes, add them into teriyaki sauce, toss until well coated and marinate for 10 minutes.

3. When ready to cook, take a grill pan, place it over medium-high heat, grease it with oil, and when hot, add marinated eggplant.

4. Cook for 3 to 4 minutes per side until nicely browned and beginning to charred, drizzling with excess marinade frequently and transfer to a plate.

5. Sprinkle green onion on top of the eggplant and then serve.

6. Meal Prep Instructions:

7. Cool the eggplant, divide evenly between two meal prep containers, and cover with a lid and then store the containers in the refrigerator for up to 7 days. When ready to eat, reheat soup in the microwave oven for 1 to 2 minutes until hot and then serve.

Nutrition: Calories 132 Fats; 4 g Protein; 13.2 g Carb; 4g

13. Scalloped Potatoes

Preparation time: 10 minutes

Cooking time: 30 minutes

Servings: 1

Ingredients:

- 1 1/3 tablespoon flour
- 3 potatoes, peeled, sliced
- 2 green onions, sliced
- 6 tablespoons almond milk, unsweetened
- 3 tablespoons grated parmesan cheese

Extra:

- ¼ teaspoon salt
- ¼ teaspoon ground black pepper

Directions:

1. Switch on the oven, then set it to 350 degrees F and let it preheat.
2. Meanwhile, take a small saucepan, place it over medium-low heat, add butter and when it melts, stir in flour until smooth sauce comes together and then stir in salt and black pepper. Whisk in milk until smooth, then remove the pan from heat and stir in 2 tablespoons cheese until melted.
3. Take a baking pan, grease it with oil, line its bottom with some of the potato slices, and sprinkle with one-third of green onion, and cover with one-third of the sauce.

4. Create two more layers by using remaining potatoes, green onion, and sauce, and sprinkle cheese on top.

5. Cover baking pan with foil, bake for 20 minutes, uncover the pan and continue cooking for 5 minutes until the top has turned golden brown. Serve straight away.

6. Meal Prep Instructions:

7. Cool the scalloped potatoes in the baking pan completely, and then cover with cling film and in the refrigerator for up to 7 days. When ready to eat, transfer scallop potatoes to a heatproof plate, reheat in the microwave oven for 1 to 2 minutes until hot, and then serve.

Nutrition: 308 Cal 5.4 g Fats 7 g Protein 57.4 g Carb 8.1 g Fiber

14. Green Onion Stir-Fry

Preparation time: 5 minutes

Cooking time: 10 minutes

Servings: 2

Ingredients:

- 2 green onions, sliced, whites and greens separated
- 4 ounces sliced mushrooms
- ½ teaspoon minced garlic
- 1 teaspoon soy sauce
- 1 tablespoon olive oil

Extra:

- 1/3 teaspoon salt
- ¼ teaspoon ground black pepper
- ¼ teaspoon red pepper flakes

Directions:

1. Take a medium skillet pan, place it over medium heat, add oil and when hot, add half of the whites of onion and then cook for 2 minutes until softened.
2. Add remaining green onions along with garlic and mushrooms, stir well and then cook for 2 to 3 minutes until mushrooms have turned golden brown and tender.
3. Drizzle with soy sauce, sprinkle with salt, black pepper, and red pepper flakes, stir until mixed and continue cooking for 1 minute until thoroughly heated.
4. Serve straight away.
5. Meal Prep Instructions:
6. Cool the mushrooms divide evenly between two meal prep containers, cover with a lid, and then store the containers in the refrigerator for up to 7 days. When ready to eat, reheat mushrooms in the microwave oven for 1 to 2 minutes until hot and then serve.

Nutrition: 81 Cal 6.8 g Fats 1.4 g Protein 2.7 g Carb 0.8 g Fiber

15. Sautéed Carrot and Green Onions

Servings: 2

Preparation time: 5 minutes;

Cooking time: 15 minutes;

Ingredients:

- 4 carrots, peeled, sliced in rounds
- 2 green onions, diced
- ½ teaspoon salt
- ¾ tablespoon olive oil
- ½ tablespoon butter, unsalted

Extra:

- ¼ teaspoon ground black pepper

Directions:

1. Take a medium bowl, fill it half full with water, add some ice, and set aside until required.
2. Take a medium saucepan, place it over medium heat, fill it half full with water, add 2/3 teaspoon salt, stir until mixed and bring it to a rolling boil.
3. Then add carrot slices, cook them for 3 to 5 minutes, don't overcook and then transfer them to the bowl containing ice-chilled water.
4. Let carrots soak until cooled and then pat dry.
5. Take a medium skillet pan, place it over medium heat, add oil and butter and wait until butter melts.

6. Then add carrot sliced and cook for 3 to 5 minutes per side until golden brown.

7. Add green onions, stir until mixed and cook for another minute.

8. Season carrots with salt and black pepper and serve.

9. Meal Prep Instructions:

10. Cool the carrots and green onions, divide evenly between two meal prep containers, and cover with a lid and then store the containers in the refrigerator for up to 7 days. When ready to eat, reheat in the microwave oven for 1 to 2 minutes until hot and then serve.

Nutrition: 123.5 Cal 8.1 g Fats 1 g Protein 11.7 g Carb 3.7 g Fiber

16. Chickpeas and Rice

Preparation time: 5 minutes

Cooking time: 15 minutes

Servings: 2

Ingredients:

- 1 tomato, chopped
- 6 ounces canned chickpeas, liquid reserved
- 10 ounces of brown rice
- 1 tablespoon olive oil
- 2/3 teaspoon salt

Extra:

- 1/3 teaspoon ground black pepper
- ½ teaspoon red pepper flakes
- ½ teaspoon cumin seeds
- Water as needed

Directions:

1. Take a medium skillet pan, add oil and when hot, add tomatoes, stir and cook for 2 to 3 minutes until softened.
2. Then add salt, black pepper, red pepper, and cumin, stir until mixed and cook for 1 minute.
3. Pour reserved chickpea liquid in a cup and add water so that liquid is 1 2/3 cup.
4. Add chickpeas into the pan, stir until coated, cook for 1 minute, then pour in the liquid and bring it to a simmer.
5. Then add rice, switch heat to medium-low heat and cook for 4 to 5 minutes until water is absorbed by rice and rice have turned tender. When done, fluff rice with a fork and then serve.
6. Meal Prep Instructions:
7. Cool the rice thoroughly, divide evenly between two meal prep containers, and cover with a lid and then store the containers in the refrigerator for up to 7 days. Reheat in the microwave oven for 1 to 2 minutes until hot when ready to eat.

Nutrition: 709 Cal;13.4 g Fats; 14.2 g Protein; 133 g Carb; 11.3 g Fiber

17. Potatoes and Mushrooms

Preparation time: 5 minutes
Cooking time: 15 minutes
Servings: 2

Ingredients:
- 8 ounces diced potato
- 4 ounces sliced mushrooms
- ½ teaspoon garlic powder
- 1 tablespoon olive oil
- 3 tablespoons almond milk, unsweetened

Extra:
- ¼ teaspoon salt
- 1/8 teaspoon ground black pepper
- 2 tablespoons water

Directions:
1. Take a medium skillet pan, place it over medium heat, add oil and when hot, add mushrooms, stir in garlic powder and cook for 5 minutes.
2. Stir in water, then add potatoes, season with salt and black pepper and continue cooking for 5 minutes or more until potatoes have cooked.
3. Switch heat to the low level, stir in milk, and then simmer for 5 to 7 minutes until vegetables have thoroughly cooked. Serve straight away.
4. Meal Prep Instructions:
5. Cool the potatoes and mushrooms, divide evenly between two meal prep containers, and cover with a lid and then store the containers in the refrigerator for up to 7 days. Reheat in the microwave oven for 1 to 2 minutes when ready to eat.

Nutrition: 158 Cal; 7 g Fats; 3.2 g Protein; 20.5 g Carb; 2.7 g Fiber

18. Parmesan and Wine Tilapia

Preparation time: 10 minutes

Cooking time: 15 minutes

Servings: 2

Ingredients:

- 1/4 C. all-purpose flour
- 1/2 C. grated Parmesan cheese
- 1/2 tsp. dried thyme
- 1/2 tsp. dried dill weed
- 1/4 tsp. salt
- 1/2 C. milk
- 1/2 C. all-purpose flour
- 4 (4 oz.) tilapia fillets
- 2 tbsps. Butter
- 1/4 C. dry white wine
- 1/4 C. milk

Directions:

1. Get a bowl, combine: salt, a quarter of a C. of flour, dill, parmesan, and thyme.
2. Get a 2nd bowl and add in 1/2 C. of flour.
3. Get a 3rd bowl and add in 1/2 a C. of milk.
4. Coat your fish with the contents of the 2nd bowl, then the 3rd bowl, and finally with the contents of the 1st bowl.
5. For 3 minutes each side brown the tilapia in butter.

6. Now set the heat to low and cook everything for 4 more minutes. Then place the fish to the side.

7. Turn up the heat and add the first bowl (flour with spices) to the pan.

8. Pour in the wine and cook the mix for 7 minutes until it becomes sauce-like.

9. Slowly stir in a quarter of a C. of milk over a low heat and cook everything for 3 more minutes.

10. Top your fish with the sauce.

11. Enjoy.

Nutrition: Calories 324 kcal Fat 11.2 g Carbohydrates 20.8g Protein 30.8 g Cholesterol 69 mg Sodium 409 mg

19. Easy Baked Tilapia

Preparation time: 20 minutes

Cooking time: 20 minutes

Servings: 8

Ingredients:

- Cooking spray
- 1/2 C. milk
- 1/2 C. prepared ranch dressing
- 1/2 C. all-purpose flour
- 1 C. dry bread crumbs
- 1/2 C. grated Parmesan cheese
- 1/2 tsp. seasoned salt
- 1/2 tsp. ground black pepper
- 1/2 tsp. celery salt
- 1/2 tsp. garlic powder
- 1/2 tsp. onion powder
- 1/2 tsp. ground paprika
- 1/2 tsp. dried parsley
- 1/4 tsp. dried basil
- Cooking spray
- 8 (6 oz.) tilapia fillets

Directions:

1. Set your oven to 425 degrees before doing anything else.

2. Cover a casserole dish with foil and then coat it with nonstick spray.

3. Get a bowl, combine: milk and the dressing.

4. Get a 2nd bowl for your flour.

5. Get a 3rd bowl, combine: parsley, bread crumbs, basil, parmesan, paprika, seasoned salt, onion powder, black pepper, and celery salt.

6. Now coat this mix with some nonstick spray until it is slightly moist. Then stir the mix a few times.

7. Do these 3 more times (spray then stir).

8. Now pour this mix in a plastic bag that can be resealed.

9. Coat your fish with the contents of the 2nd bowl, then the 1st bowl, and finally put each piece individually into your plastic bag and shake everything to coat the fish.

10. Place your fish pieces in the casserole dish and coat them with a little more cooking spray.

11. Cook everything in the oven for 23 minutes.

12. Enjoy.

Nutrition: Calories 357 kcal Fat 12.8 g Carbohydrates 17.8g Protein 39.8 g Cholesterol 71 mg Sodium 550 mg

20. Butter, Garlic, and Tomatoes Tilapia

Preparation time: 10 minutes

Cooking time: 15 minutes

Servings: 4

Ingredients:

- 4 (4 oz.) fillets tilapia
- Salt and pepper to taste
- 4 tbsps. Butter
- 3 cloves garlic, pressed
- 4 fresh basil leaves, diced
- 1 large tomato, diced
- 1 C. white wine

Directions:

- Get an outdoor grill hot and coat the grate with some oil before doing anything else.
- Now lay all your pieces of fish on a big piece of foil.
- Coat each piece with pepper and salt then put 1 tbsp. of butter on each one.
- Now top each piece with tomato, basil, and garlic. Then cover everything with the wine.
- Wrap some foil around the fish and seal it tightly.
- Place the foiled fish in a casserole dish and bring everything over to the grill.
- Grill your fish for 17 minutes.
- Enjoy.

Nutrition: Calories 277 kcal Fat 13.1 g Carbohydrates 4.2g Protein 23.7 g Cholesterol 72 mg Sodium 159 mg

21. Spicy Garlic Tilapia

Preparation time: 5 minutes

Cooking time: 30 minutes

Servings: 4

Ingredients:

- 4 (4 oz.) fillets tilapia
- 4 cloves crushed garlic
- 3 tbsps. Olive oil
- 1 onion, diced
- 1/4 tsp. cayenne pepper

Directions:

1. Take your pieces of garlic and rub the pieces of fish with it. Now place everything into a casserole dish.
2. Coat your tilapia with olive oil and then layer your onions over everything.
3. Place a covering around the dish and place everything in the fridge for 8 hrs.
4. Set your oven to 350 degrees before doing anything else.
5. Top your fish with the cayenne and cook everything in the oven for 32 minutes.
6. Enjoy.

Nutrition: Calories 217 kcal Fat 11.7 g Carbohydrates 3.6g
Protein 23.5 g Cholesterol 41 mg Sodium 74 mg

22. Salmon with Baby Arugula

Preparation Time: 25 minutes

Cooking time: 10 minutes

Servings: 2

Ingredients:

- Salmon (2 center cut filets)
- Olive oil (1 ½ tablespoons)
- Black pepper
- Lemon juice (1 ½ tablespoons)
- All purpose seasoning (1/8 teaspoon)

For salad:

- Cherry tomatoes (2/3 cup, cut in half)
- Black pepper
- Wine vinegar (1 tablespoon)
- Baby arugula (3 cups)
- Red onion (1/4 cup, sliced)
- Olive oil (1 tablespoon, extra virgin)

Directions:

1. Season fish with all purpose, oil and lemon juice; marinate for 15 minutes.
2. Heat skillet and place the salmon onto the skin side into the pot and cook for 3 minutes. Use a spatula to lightly lift fish to avoid sticking.
3. Lower heat and cover pan; cook for 4 minutes until skin is crispy.
4. Combine onion, tomatoes and arugula in a bowl then drizzle with vinegar and oil.
5. Serve salad with fish.

Nutrition: Calories 390 Carbs 4g Fat 23g Protein 40g

23. Baked Cod & Green Beans

Preparation Time: 30 minutes

Cooking time: 15 minutes

Servings: 1

Ingredients:

- Olive oil (2 teaspoons)
- Cod (4 oz.)
- Green beans (2 cups)
- Blueberries (1/2 cup)
- Old-fashioned oats (1 tablespoon)
- Tomato (2 slices)

Directions:

1. Set oven to 400°F.
2. Combine oats and half of oil in a bowl and use mixture to coat fish.
3. Coat baking tray with cooking spray and place fish onto tray and top with the tomato slices and bake for 15 minutes.
4. Steam green beans and serve with fish and blueberries.

Nutrition: Calories 350 Carbs 39g Fat 11g Protein 27g

24. Baked Scallops

Preparation Time: 30 minutes

Cooking time: 10 minutes

Servings: 1

Ingredients:

- Bay scallops (3 oz.)
- Oats (1 tablespoon, old-fashioned)
- Olive oil (1 ½ teaspoons, extra-virgin)
- Lemon pepper
- Garbanzo beans (1/4 cup, low salt)
- Cucumber (1 cup)
- White wine (3 tablespoons)
- Cheddar cheese (1/2 oz., low fat, shredded)
- Lemon juice (3 tablespoons, freshly squeezed)
- Romaine lettuce (3 cups, chopped)
- Tomato (1)

Directions:

1. Put scallops into a container and cover with white wine; cover container and put into refrigerator overnight.
2. Set oven to 350°F.
3. Remove scallops from wine and top with oats and cheese.
4. Place onto a baking tray and bake for 10 minutes.
5. Combine lemon pepper, lemon juice and oil in a small bowl.
6. Mix together garbanzo beans, cucumber, lettuce and tomato.
7. Serve salad topped with lemon dressing and baked scallops.

Nutrition: Calories 358 Carbs 34g Fat 11g Protein 27g

25. Indian Inspired Filet Of Fish Ii

Preparation time: 20 minutes

Cooking time: 35 minutes

Servings: 4

Ingredients:

Marinade:

- 2 tsps Dijon mustard
- 1 tsp ground black pepper
- 1/2 tsp salt
- 2 tbsps canola oil
- 4 white fish fillets
- 1 onion, coarsely chopped
- 4 cloves garlic, roughly chopped
- 1 (1 inch) piece fresh ginger root, peeled and chopped
- 5 cashew halves
- 1 tbsp canola oil
- 2 tsps cayenne pepper, or to taste
- 1/2 tsp ground turmeric
- 1 tsp ground cumin
- 1 tsp ground coriander
- 1 tsp salt
- 1 tsp white sugar
- 1/2 C. chopped tomato
- 1/4 C. vegetable broth
- 1/4 C. chopped fresh cilantro

Directions

1. Set your oven at 350 degrees F before doing anything else.
2. Coat fish fillets with a mixture of mustard, pepper, 1/2 tsp salt, and 2 tbsps of canola oil before refrigerating it for 30 minutes.
3. Cook blended mixture of onion, cashews, ginger and garlic for two minutes before adding cayenne pepper, 1 tsp salt, turmeric, cumin, coriander and sugar in the pan, and cooking it for 5 more minutes.
4. Add chopped tomato and vegetable broth before pouring it over the fish in the baking dish.
5. Bake this in the preheated oven for about 30 minutes.
6. Sprinkle some chopped cilantro for garnishing.

Nutrition: Calories 338 kcal Carbohydrates 11.6 g Cholesterol 56 mg Fat 13.5 g Fiber 2.3 g Protein 41.6 g Sodium 2715 mg

26. Orzo and Spiced Shrimp

Preparation Time: 40 minutes

Cooking time: 10 minutes

Servings: 2

Ingredients:

- Orzo pasta (2/3 cup)
- Olive oil (1 tablespoon)
- Black pepper
- Chile powder (1/2 teaspoon, ancho)
- Cumin (1/4 teaspoon)
- Cayenne pepper
- Lime juice (3 tablespoons, freshly squeezed)
- Red onion (1/2, sliced)
- Basil leaves (2 tablespoons)
- Smoked paprika (1 teaspoon)
- Agave nectar (1 teaspoon)
- Coriander (1/4 teaspoon)
- Jumbo shrimp (3 oz., deveined and without shell)
- Lettuce (8 leaves)
- Tomatoes (2, sliced)

Directions:

1. Put oil and basil into a processor or blender and pulse until smooth. Add black pepper and lime juice, mx together and put aside until needed.

2. Heat grill.

3. Combine chili powder, cumin, cayenne pepper, paprika, sugar and coriander in a small bowl.

4. Coat shrimp with cooking spray and spice blend and put aside; prepare orzo as directed on package, run under cold water and drain.

5. Pour lime juice over orzo.

6. Grill shrimp for 4 minutes until slightly charred.

7. Place lettuce on a place and top with orzo, onion and tomato and drizzle with basil blend.

8. Add shrimp and serve.

Nutrition: Calories 345 Carbs 35g Fat 11g Protein 26g

27. Apple Scallops

Preparation Time: 15 minutes

Cooking time: 5 minutes

Servings: 1

Ingredients:

- Celery (3/4 cup, diced)
- Vegetable broth (1/2 cup, no salt)
- Ginger (1/2 teaspoon, grated)
- Cardamom (1 teaspoon)
- Olive oil (1 teaspoon)
- Carrot (1/3 cup, shredded)
- Green beans (1 cup)
- Green apple (3/4, without core and chopped)
- Scallops (4 oz.)
- Walnuts (1 tablespoon, crushed)

Directions:

1. Add carrots and celery to pot along with 3 tablespoon broth and cook for 5 minutes.
2. Put in leftover broth along with ginger, cardamom, green beans and apple; mix together to combine and cook until thoroughly heated.
3. Heat skillet and coat with cooking spray and cook scallops on all sides until golden.
4. Serve with vegetables and top with walnuts and olive oil.

Nutrition: Calories 324 Carbs 36g Fat 11g Protein 23g

28. Easy Little Fish Tacos

Preparation time: 20 minutes

Cooking time: 30 minutes

Servings: 8

Ingredients:

- 1 pound shark fillets
- 12 (6 inch) corn tortillas
- 1/4 cup canola oil
- 1/4 cup lemon juice
- 1 clove garlic, minced
- 1 teaspoon dried oregano
- 1 teaspoon Cajun seasoning
- 1 cup shredded Cheddar cheese
- 2 quarts vegetable oil for frying

Directions:

1. Coat shark strips with a mixture of canola oil, oregano, lemon juice, garlic and Cajun style spice mix, and marinate it for at least an hour before placing each one of them on microwaved tortillas.

2. Fold it up and seal it up with a toothpick before frying it up for 4 minutes.

3. Place all these tortillas on the baking dish and bake at 350 degrees F for five minutes.

4. Serve.

Nutrition: Calories 642 kcal Carbohydrates 25.1 g Cholesterol 55 mg Fat 51.3 g Fiber 3.5 g Protein 22.4 g Sodium 295 mg

29. Easy Deep Fried Snapper

Preparation time: 5 minutes

Cooking time: 10 minutes

Servings: 4

Ingredients:

- 1 quart vegetable oil for frying
- 1 lb red snapper fillets
- 1 egg, beaten
- 1/2 C. dry bread crumbs

Directions:

1. Dip fish fillets in beaten egg before dipping in the bread crumbs.
2. Fry these fillets in hot oil until you see that it is golden brown.
3. Serve.

Nutrition: Calories 386 kcal Carbohydrates 9.8 g Cholesterol 92 mg Fat 26.2 g Fiber 0.6 g Protein 26.8 g Sodium 175 mg

30. Louisiana Style Mahi Mahi

Preparation time: 10 minutes

Cooking time: 20 minutes

Servings: 2

Ingredients:

- 2 (4 oz.) fillets mahi mahi
- 2 tsps olive oil
- 1/2 C. salted butter
- 1 clove garlic, minced
- 1 tbsp lemon juice
- 2 drops Louisiana-style hot sauce, or to taste
- 1 roma tomato, seeded and chopped (optional)
- 1 green onion, chopped

Directions:

1. Set your oven at 450 degrees F before doing anything else.
2. Coat mahi mahi fillets with olive oil and place them in the baking dish
3. Bake this in the preheated oven for about 20 minutes.
4. Cook garlic, lemon juice and hot sauce in hot butter for one minute before adding tomato and green onion.
5. Continue cooking for another 3 minutes before pouring it over the baked fish.

Nutrition: Calories 556 kcal Carbohydrates 3 g Cholesterol 204 mg Fat 51.7 g Fiber 0.6 g Protein 21.7 g Sodium 452 mg

31. Indian Style Tandoori Catfish

Serving: 6

Preparation time: 10 minutes

Cooking time: 17 minutes

Ingredients:

- 1/3 C. vinegar
- 4 cloves garlic
- 1 tbsp chopped fresh ginger
- 1/2 tsp salt
- 1 tbsp cayenne pepper
- 1 tbsp ground coriander
- 1 tbsp ground cumin
- 1/2 C. vegetable oil
- 2 lbs thick catfish fillets, cut into large chunks

Directions:

1. Coat fish chunks with a mixture of vinegar, cayenne, garlic, ginger, salt, coriander, cumin, and oil before marinating it for at least four hours.
2. Heat up the broiler.
3. Now broil the fish in the preheated broiler for about 10 minutes before turning and brushing it with the reserved marinade.
4. Broil for another 7 minutes.
5. Serve.

Nutrition: Calories 272 kcal Carbohydrates 2.3 g Cholesterol 71 mg Fat 30.2 g Fiber 0.9 g Protein 24.1 g Sodium 277 mg

32. Easy Jalapeno Garlic Trout

Preparation time: 10 minutes

Cooking time: 20 minutes

Servings: 2

Ingredients:

- 2 rainbow trout fillets
- 1 tbsp olive oil
- 2 tsps garlic salt
- 1 tsp ground black pepper
- 1 fresh jalapeno pepper, sliced
- 1 lemon, sliced

Directions:

1. Set your oven at 400 degrees F before doing anything else.
2. Coat fillets with olive oil, black pepper and garlic salt before putting jalapeno slices, lemon juice and lemon slices over fillets in some aluminum foil.
3. Wrap these foils up before placing them in a baking dish.
4. Bake in the preheated oven for about 20 minutes.

Nutrition: Calories 213 kcal Carbohydrates 7.5 g Cholesterol 67 mg Fat 10.9 g Fiber 3 g Protein 24.3 g Sodium 1850 mg

33. Veracruz Scallops with Green Chile Sauce

Preparation time:20 minutes

Cooking Time: 20 minutes

Servings: 8 persons

Ingredients

- 24 (2 ounces) sea scallops, large pieces
- Finely grated juice and zest of 1 lime, fresh
- Vegetable oil, as required

For Rub

- 1 teaspoon pure chile powder
- ½ teaspoon ground cumin
- 1 teaspoon paprika
- ½ teaspoon oregano, dried
- 1 teaspoon kosher salt
- ¼ teaspoon freshly ground black pepper

For Sauce

- 3 long Anaheim chile peppers
- ½ cup sour cream
- 3 scallions (green and white parts only), coarsely chopped
- ½ cup mayonnaise
- 1 garlic clove, small
- ¼ cup fresh cilantro leaves & tender stems; loosely packed
- Finely grated juice & zest of 1 lime, fresh
- ¼ teaspoon kosher salt

Directions:

1. Preheat the grill over high heat for direct cooking
2. Grill the chile peppers for a couple of minutes, until turn blackened & blistered in spots, with the lid open, turning every now and then. Remove the chiles from grill; set aside until easy

to handle. Once done; remove the stem ends & discard. Scrape off & discard the blackened skins using a sharp knife. Coarsely chop the leftover parts of chiles & drop them into a blender or food processor. Add the scallions followed by garlic, and cilantro. Process on high power until you get coarse paste like consistency; scraping down the sides of your bowl as required. Add the leftover sauce ingredients & process on high power again until you get smooth sauce.

3. Next, mix the entire rub ingredients together in a small-sized mixing bowl.

4. Rinse the scallops under cold running tap water & remove the tough, small muscle. Place the cleaned scallops in a large-sized mixing bowl & add oil (enough to coat). Add the rub mixture followed by the lime juice, and lime zest. Mix well until the scallops are evenly coated.

5. Grill the scallops for 4 to 6 minutes, until opaque in the middle and firm slightly on the surface, with the lid closed, turning once. Remove from the grill; serve warm with the prepared sauce and enjoy.

Nutrition: 208 Calories 182 Calories from Fat 20g Total Fat 4.3g Saturated Fat 0.3g Trans Fat 10g Polyunsaturated Fat 4.6g Monounsaturated Fat 22mg Cholesterol 698mg Sodium 168mg Potassium 5g Total Carbohydrates 0.9g Dietary Fiber 2.3g Sugars 2.4g Protein

34. Grilled Fresh Fish

Preparation Time: 10 Minutes

Cooking Time: 25 Minutes

Servings: 4 Persons

Ingredients:

- 1 whole firm white fish fillet: such as halibut, sea bass or cod
- 2 whole lemons; sliced into half
- Traeger Fin & Feather Rub, as required

Directions:

1. Preheat your wood pellet to 325 F in advance for 12 to 15 minutes, lid closed.
2. Season the fish with Rub & let sit for half an hour.
3. Place the fish & lemons directly over the hot grill grates, cut side down. Cook until the fish is flaky, for 12 to 15 minutes. Ensure that you don't overcook the fish. Serve immediately with grilled lemons and enjoy.

Nutrition: 30 Calories 2.5 Calories from Fat 0.3g Total Fat 0.1g Saturated Fat 0g Trans Fat 0.1g Polyunsaturated Fat 0g Monounsaturated Fat 16mg Cholesterol 20mg Sodium 146mg Potassium 3.9g Total Carbohydrates 1.2g Dietary Fiber 1.1g Sugars 4.4g Protein

35. Sanibel Southern Style

Preparation Time: 10 minutes

Cooking time: 15

Servings: 4

Ingredients:

- 1 tbsp. olive oil
- Salt and pepper to taste
- 2 (8 oz.) steaks halibut
- 3 tbsp. capers, with liquid
- 1/2 C. white wine
- 1 tsp. chopped garlic
- 1/4 C. butter

Directions:

1. heat the olive oil on medium-high heat and fry the halibut steaks in a large skillet, till browned from all sides.
2. Transfer the steaks into a bowl and keep aside.
3. In the same pan, add the wine and with a spatula scrape any browned bits from the bottom.
4. Cook till the wine is almost absorbed.
5. Stir in the garlic, butter, capers, salt and pepper and simmer for 1 minute.
6. Stir in the steaks and cook till the fish flakes easily with a fork.

Nutrition: Calories 284 kcal Fat 17 g Carbohydrates 1.4g Protein 24.2 g Cholesterol 72 mg Sodium 337

36. Halibut

Preparation Time: 10 minutes

Cooking time: 25 minutes

Servings: 4

Ingredients:

- 2 lb. halibut steak, 1 1/2-inch thickness
- 1/4 tsp. ground white pepper
- 1 C. sour cream
- 1 pinch dried dill weed
- 1/2 C. chopped green onions
- 1/3 C. grated Parmesan cheese
- 2 tbsp. butter, softened
- 1/2 tsp. salt

Directions:

1. Before doing anything else, set your oven to 350 degrees F and grease a 13x9-inch baking dish with the butter.
2. Arrange the halibut steak in the prepared baking dish.
3. In a bowl, mix together the sour cream, green onions, butter, salt, white pepper and dill.
4. Place the sour cream mixture over the halibut steak evenly. Cook in the oven for about 20-25 minutes.
5. Bring out the halibut from the oven and sprinkle with the Parmesan cheese.
6. Now, set your oven to broiler and arrange oven rack about 6-inches from the heating element.
7. Cook the fish under the broiler for about 2-3 minutes.

Nutrition: Calories 461 kcal Fat 24 g Carbohydrates 3.9g Protein 53.3 g Cholesterol 131 mg Sodium 593 mg

37. Restaurant Style Halibut

Preparation Time: 15 minutes

Cooking time: 35 minutes

Servings: 6

Ingredients:

- 2 lb. halibut fillets
- 1 (16 oz.) can diced tomatoes
- Salt and pepper to taste
- 2 tbsp. capers
- 1/4 C. olive oil
- 4 cloves garlic, minced
- 1/2 C. chopped fresh parsley
- 1 yellow onion, thinly sliced
- 2 stalks celery, chopped
- 1 green bell pepper, chopped

Directions:

1. Before doing anything else, set your oven to 475 degrees F and lightly, grease a 13x9-inch baking dish.
2. Wash the halibut and pat dry with the paper towels.
3. Cut the halibut into serving size pieces 4. Arrange the halibut pieces into prepared baking dish and sprinkle with the salt and pepper.
4. Mix together the olive oil, parsley, onion, celery, bell pepper, tomatoes, capers and garlic in a bowl, .

5. Place the oil mixture over the halibut pieces evenly.

6. Cook in the oven for about 20 minutes.

7. Remove from the oven and keep aside for about 10 minutes before serving.

Nutrition: Calories 291 kcal Fat 12 g Carbohydrates 8.5g Protein 34 g Cholesterol 56 mg Sodium 304 mg

38. Whangarei Style

Preparation Time: 20 minutes

Cooking time: 25 minutes

Servings: 4

Ingredients:

- 1 tbsp. butter
- 1/2 tsp. red pepper flakes
- 1 tbsp. olive oil
- 1 lb. mussels, cleaned and debearded
- 2 tbsp. minced garlic
- 1 C. chopped green onions
- 2 tbsp. minced shallots
- 1 tbsp. capers
- 3 C. canned tomato sauce
- 1 tbsp. Italian seasoning

Directions:

1. Heat the oil and butter on medium temperature in a skillet and sauté the shallots, garlic and capers for about 5 minutes .
2. Stir in the Italian herbs, tomato sauce and red pepper flakes and reduce the heat to medium-low.
3. Simmer, covered for about 10 minutes.
4. Stir in the mussels and increase the heat to medium-high.
5. Cook, covered for about 10 minutes.
6. Discard any unopened mussels from the skillet.
7. Serve with a garnishing of the green onions.

Nutrition: Calories 142 kcal Fat 7.1 g Carbohydrates 15.8g Protein 6.9 g Cholesterol 17 mg Sodium 1102 mg

39. French Mussels

Preparation Time: 20 minutes

Cooking time: 20 minutes

Servings: 4

Ingredients:

- 2 tbsp. butter
- 20 fresh basil leaves, torn
- 3 tbsp. minced garlic
- 2 C. white wine
- 4 shallots, chopped
- 1 tbsp. cornstarch
- 4 C. beef broth
- 1/2 C. light cream
- 1 jalapeno pepper, minced
- 5 lb. fresh mussels, scrubbed and
- 1 red chili pepper, minced
- Debearded
- 4 fresh tomatoes, coarsely chopped

Directions:

1. Melt the butter on medium temperature in a large soup pan, and sauté the shallots and garlic till browned lightly.

2. Add the red chile pepper, jalapeño and a splash of the broth and simmer for a few minutes.

3. Stir in the remaining broth, white wine, tomatoes and basil and bring to a boil.

4. Meanwhile in a bowl, mix together the cornstarch and a little amount of the light cream.

5. In the pan, add the remaining light cream and cornstarch mixture and bring to a boil.

6. Cook for about 5 minutes.

Nutrition: Calories 413 kcal Fat 13.8 g Carbohydrates 27.2g Protein 24 g Cholesterol 80 mg Sodium 1109 mg

Pescatarian Soups

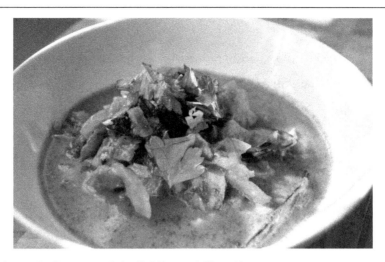

40. Spinach Soup with Dill and Basil

Preparation time: 10 minutes

Cooking time: 25 minutes

Servings: 8

Ingredients:

- 1 pound peeled and diced potatoes
- 1 tablespoon minced garlic
- 1 teaspoon dry mustard
- 6 cups vegetable broth
- 20 ounces chopped frozen spinach
- 2 cups chopped onion
- 1 ½ tablespoons salt
- ½ cup minced dill
- 1 cup basil

- ½ teaspoon ground black pepper

Directions:

1. Whisk onion, garlic, potatoes, broth, mustard, and salt in a pan and cook it over medium flame. When it starts boiling, low down the heat and covers it with the lid and cook for 20 minutes. Add the remaining ingredients in it and blend it and cook it for few more minutes and serve it.

Nutrition: Carbohydrates 12g, Protein 13g, Fats 1g, Calories 165

41. Miyeokguk - Korean Seaweed Soup with mussels

Preparation time: 20 minutes

Cooking time: 45 minutes

Servings: 6-8

Ingredients:

- 1 ounce dried miyeok, soaked in cold water for 30 minutes
- 2 pounds fresh mussels, cleaned, rinsed, and drained
- 4 cloves garlic, minced
- 8 cups of water
- 2 tablespoons fish sauce
- 3 teaspoons sesame oil
- 4 green onions, chopped
- Salt to taste

Directions:

1. Place the mussels in a large bowl and cover them with cold water. Mix in 1 tablespoon of salt making it into brine. Soak for 30 minutes so that the mussels let out any dirt or sand. Drain and rinse well in cold water. At the same time, place miyeok in cold water and let soak for 30 minutes. Drain, rinse, and squeeze out any excess water. Chop the miyeok a bit to make it into bite sized pieces.

2. In a large soup pot, add 8 cups of water and place the miyeok into the water. Cook covered on medium heat for 20 to 25 minutes until the miyeok turns soft and the water is infused with its flavor.

3. Add the mussels, garlic, fish sauce and stir gently. Cover and cook for about 15 minutes over medium high heat. The mussels will now open up they will release flavor into the broth. Remove the soup from the heat, drizzle the sesame oil in. Ladle the soup into serving bowls and garnish with green onion.

4. Serve with rice, kimchi, and possibly more Korean side dishes.

Nutrition: Calories: 89

42. Hot and Sour Soup With Shrimp with lemongrass

Preparation time: 20 minutes

Cooking time: 35 minutes

Servings: 4-6

Ingredients:

- 2 tablespoons coconut oil
- 3/4 pound shiitake mushrooms, stemmed, caps sliced 1/4th inch think
- 4 Thai chilies, minced
- 3 stalks of fresh lemongrass, inner bulbs only, thinly sliced
- 1-pound medium shrimp, shelled and deveined, shells reserved
- 1 large onion, chopped
- 1/2 cup thinly sliced fresh ginger
- 1/4-cup Asian fish sauce
- 8 cups fresh vegetable stock
- 1/4-cup fresh lime juice
- 1/2-cup small basil leaves
- Salt and freshly ground black pepper to taste

Directions:

1. In a large, deep skillet, heat 1 tablespoon of the oil. Add shiitake mushrooms and season with salt and pepper. Cover and cook over medium heat, stirring occasionally, until tender, 5 minutes. Uncover and cook, stirring, until the mushrooms are golden, about 3 minutes. Transfer to a plate.

2. Add the remaining 1-tablespoon of oil to the skillet. Add the chilies lemongrass, shrimp shells, onion, and ginger and cover over medium heat, stirring occasionally, until the onion is

softened and golden brown, about 7 minutes. Add the fish sauce and fresh stock and bring to a boil. Simmer over medium heat for 10 minutes, strain in a large bowl.

3. Return the broth to the skillet; bring to a simmer over medium heat. Add the shrimp, mushrooms, and cook until the shrimp are pink and curled, about 1 minute. Add the lime juice and season with salt and pepper. Ladle the soup into bowls, garnish with basil leaves and serve.

Nutrition: Calories: 99

43. Manhattan Clam Chowder

Preparation time: 20 minutes

Cooking time: 30 minutes

Servings: 6-8

Ingredients:

- 8 pounds large cherrystone clams, scrubbed and rinsed, opened clams discarded
- 4 tablespoons coconut oil
- 2 large onions, finely chopped
- 2 stalks celery, finely chopped
- 1 bell pepper, chopped
- 1 large carrot, diced
- 3 cloves garlic, minced
- 3 bay leaves
- 1 1/2 teaspoons dried oregano leaves
- 4 sprigs fresh thyme
- 1/2 teaspoon crushed red pepper
- 5 medium Idaho potatoes cut into 1/2-inch cubes
- 1-cup fresh vegetable broth
- 6 medium ripe tomatoes, seeded and chopped, juice reserved
- 1/4 cup parsley leaves, chopped
- Kosher salt and freshly ground black pepper to taste

Directions:

1. In a large stockpot, bring 2 cups of water to a boil. Add clams, cover and cook for 5 minutes. Uncover, stir clams well with a wooden spoon and cover. Allow clams to cook 5-8 minutes longer (depending on the size of the clams and type) or until most of the clams have opened. Transfer clams to a large bowl and strain broth through a fine-meshed sieve into a bowl. (There should be about 6 cups of clam broth. If not add some water to bring it the volume to 6 cups.) When clams are cool enough to handle, remove them from their shells and chop into 1/2-inch pieces. Set clams and broth aside.

2. In a large heavy pot on medium heat, heat coconut oil. Add onions, celery, bell pepper and carrots and cook for 10 minutes, until vegetables are softened. Add garlic, bay leaves, oregano, thyme and crushed red pepper and cook an additional 2 minutes. Increase heat to high and add potatoes, reserved clam broth, and vegetable stock and bring to a boil, covered. Cook for 20 minutes, or until potatoes are tender and the broth has slightly thickened. Add tomatoes and continue to cook for 10 - 15 minutes. Remove the pot from heat and add reserved clams and parsley and season with salt and pepper, to taste. Allow chowder to sit for about 1 hour to allow flavors to meld, and then reheat slowly over low heat if necessary. Do not bring to boil. Serve warm/hot.

Nutrition: Calories: 159

44. Crab Bisque Soup - France

Preparation time: 15 minutes

Cooking time: 50 minutes

Servings: 6-8

Ingredients:

- 4 Dungeness crabs
- 3 tablespoons coconut oil
- 1 carrot, chopped
- 2 stalks celery, chopped
- 3 tomatoes, chopped
- 5 garlic cloves, chopped
- 5 shallots, chopped
- 3 sprigs fresh tarragon leaves, chopped
- 3 tablespoons Cognac
- 2 cups good dry white wine
- 2 tablespoons tomato paste
- 10 cups fish stock or water
- Salt to taste
- Fresh ground black pepper
- Cayenne pepper
- Pinch dried thyme
- 1 bay leaf
- 1/2-cup heavy cream
- 1 1/2 cup milk
- 1 lemon, juiced

- 1 tablespoon minced chives or parsley leaves

Directions:

1. Remove the claws from the crabs and quarter the bodies. Heat a large stockpot. Add oil and sauté the crab pieces until they are red. Remove the pieces as they are cooked. Add the carrots, celery, tomatoes, garlic, shallots, and tarragon and sauté or 10 minutes. Pour the cognac and ignite. When the flame has subsided, deglaze with white wine, and add the tomato paste, crab, and enough fish stick to cover.

2. Season it with salt, pepper, cayenne, thyme, and bay lead and boil gently for 15 minutes.

3. In a small saucepan, reduce cream and milk by half. Remove the crab bodies form the pot and set aside. Add the reduced cream to the soup. Puree the soup, in batches, in a food processor, Strain and puree soup and keep warm.

4. Remove the meat from the claws and chop it in large pieces and place it back into the soup. Add the lemon juice, salt pepper and serve hot garnished with chives and/or parsley.

Nutrition: Calories: 190

45. Cioppino - San Francisco, CA

Preparation time: 15 minutes

Cooking time: 50 minutes

Servings: 6-8

Ingredients:

- 3 tablespoons coconut oil
- 1 medium onion, chopped
- 3 medium shallots, chopped
- 2 teaspoons salt
- 4 garlic cloves, minced
- 1 teaspoon crushed red pepper flakes
- 1/4-cup tomato paste
- 1 28-ounce can diced tomatoes with juice
- 1 1/2 cups dry white wine
- 5 cups fresh seafood stock
- 2 bay leaves
- 1 pound little neck clams, scrubbed
- 1 pound mussels, scrubbed, debearded
- 1 pound fresh large shrimp, peeled and deveined
- 1 1/2 pounds assorted firm fleshed fish fillets such as cod or salmon, cut into 2 inch pieces
- 1/4 cup parsley, minced for garnish

Directions:

1. In an extra large stockpot over medium heat, heat the oil. Add the onions and shallots, and sauté, about 10 minute until translucent, season with salt and pepper. Add the garlic and pepper flakes, sauté another 2 minutes. Add tomatoes with juices and tomato paste, stir with wine and stock, and add the bay leave and cover, simmering over medium heat. Once simmer is reached, lower the heat to low and cook for 30 minutes.

2. Add the mussels and clams, cook for about 5 minutes or until they begin to open. Add the fish and shrimp, and simmer gently until the shrimp are cooked through, about 5 minutes. Make sure to discard any calms and mussels that did not open. Taste and season the soup with salt and red pepper.

3. Garnish with parsley and serve immediately.

Nutrition: Calories: 190

46. Brazilian Shrimp Soup

Preparation time: 15 minutes

Cooking time: 25 minutes

Servings: 6

Ingredients:

- 2 tablespoons coconut oil
- 1 medium onion, chopped
- 4 garlic cloves, chopped
- 1 red bell pepper, chopped
- 1/2 cup long-grain rice
- 1-2 pinches red pepper flakes (to taste)
- 2 teaspoons salt
- 1 15-ounce can crushed tomatoes
- 4 cups fresh water
- 1 cup canned unsweetened coconut milk
- 1 pound medium shrimp, shelled and cut into large pieces
- 1 lemon, juiced
- 1/2 teaspoon freshly ground black pepper
- 1/2 cup chopped fresh parsley for garnish

Directions:

1. In a large stockpot over medium heat, heat up the oil. Add onion, bell pepper, garlic, cook for about 5 minutes or until the vegetables are soft and tender. Stir frequently.

2. Add the rice, red pepper flakes, salt, tomatoes, water and bring to a boil. Cook until the rice is almost done but not quite done.

3. Add the coconut milk, stirring. Add the shrimp. Simmer, stirring occasionally until the shrimp are done, about 5 minutes. Stir in the lemon juice, black pepper. Ladle the soup into bowls and garnish with parsley to serve.

Nutrition: Calories: 183

47. Shrimp Wonton Soup

Preparation time: 20 minutes (shrimp are refrigerated overnight see below)

Cooking time: 40 minutes

Servings: 4

Ingredients:

For The Shrimp

- 1 pound shrimp, peeled, deveined, and shells reserved
- 1-teaspoon baking soda

For The Broth

- 6 cups seafood broth (shrimp broth preferred)
- 2 stalks lemongrass, peeled and crushed
- 1-inch piece ginger
- 2 green onions
- Fish sauce to taste

For The Wontons

- 1-teaspoon garlic, grated
- 1-teaspoon ginger, grated
- 2 teaspoons oyster sauce
- 1-teaspoon soy sauce
- 1/2-teaspoon sesame oil
- 1 teaspoon Shaoxing wine or dry sherry
- 1/2-teaspoon white pepper
- Wanton wrappers

For The Wonton Soup

- 2 green onions, sliced

Directions:

Shrimp:

1. Mix the baking soda into some cold water, place the shrimp into it and refrigerate overnight.

2. The Broth:

3. In a large saucepan, add broth, shrimp shells, lemongrass, ginger, and green onions to a boil. Reduce heat and simmer covered, for 1o minutes. Strain the solids, return to saucepan and season with fish sauce to taste.

The Wontons:

1. Coarsely chop the shrimp, mix with the garlic, ginger, oyster sauce, sesame oil, Shaoxing wine, and white pepper.

2. Place 2 teaspoons of the mixture into the center of a wonton wrapper with water, fold one corner over forming a triangle, seal and pull the two opposite corners along the fold back together and repeat for remaining filling.

3. Bring a pot of water to a boil, lightly salt the water, add the wontons and simmer until they float to the top.

For the Wonton Soup

4. Divide the wontons between bowls and top with the broth and garnish with green onions.

Nutrition: Calories: 175

48. Coconut Watercress Soup

Preparation time: 10 minutes

Cooking time: 20 minutes

Servings: 4

Ingredients:

- 1 teaspoon coconut oil
- 1 onion, diced
- ¾ cup coconut milk

Directions:

1. Melt the coconut oil in a large pot over medium-high heat. Add the onion and cook until soft, about 5 minutes, then add the peas and the water. Bring to a boil, then lower the heat and add the watercress, mint, salt, and pepper.

2. Cover and simmer for 5 minutes. Stir in the coconut milk and purée the soup until smooth in a blender or with an immersion blender.

3. Try this soup with any other fresh, leafy green—anything from spinach to collard greens to arugula to Swiss chard.

Nutrition: Calories: 178;Protein: 6g; Total fat: 10g; Carbohydrates: 18g; Fiber: 5g

49. Roasted Red Pepper and Butternut Squash Soup

Preparation time: 10 minutes

Cooking time: 45 minutes

Servings: 6

Ingredients:

- 1 small butternut squash
- 1 tablespoon olive oil
- 1 teaspoon sea salt
- 2 red bell peppers
- 1 yellow onion
- 1 head garlic
- 2 cups water or vegetable broth
- Zest and juice of 1 lime
- 1 to 2 tablespoons tahini
- Pinch cayenne pepper
- ½ teaspoon ground coriander
- ½ teaspoon ground cumin
- Toasted squash seeds (optional)

Directions:

1. Preparing the ingredients.
2. Preheat the oven to 350°f.
3. Prepare the squash for roasting by cutting it in half lengthwise, scooping out the seeds, and poking some holes in the flesh with a fork. Reserve the seeds if desired.
4. Rub a small amount of oil over the flesh and skin, then rub with a bit of sea salt and put the halves skin-side down in a

large baking dish. Put it in the oven while you prepare the rest of the vegetables.

5. Prepare the peppers the exact same way, except they do not need to be poked.

6. Slice the onion in half and rub oil on the exposed faces. Slice the top off the head of garlic and rub oil on the exposed flesh.

7. After the squash has cooked for 20 minutes, add the peppers, onion, and garlic, and roast for another 20 minutes. Optionally, you can toast the squash seeds by putting them in the oven in a separate baking dish 10 to 15 minutes before the vegetables are finished.

8. Keep a close eye on them. When the vegetables are cooked, take them out and let them cool before handling them. The squash will be very soft when poked with a fork.

9. Scoop the flesh out of the squash skin into a large pot (if you have an immersion blender) or into a blender.

10. Chop the pepper roughly, remove the onion skin and chop the onion roughly, and squeeze the garlic cloves out of the head, all into the pot or blender. Add the water, the lime zest and juice, and the tahini. Purée the soup, adding more water if you like, to your desired consistency. Season with the salt, cayenne, coriander, and cumin. Serve garnished with toasted squash seeds (if using).

Nutrition: Calories: 156; Protein: 4g; Total Fat: 7g; Saturated Fat: 11g; Carbohydrates: 22g; Fiber: 5g

50. Tomato Pumpkin Soup

Preparation time: 25 minutes

Cooking time: 15 minutes

Servings: 4

Ingredients:

- 2 cups pumpkin, diced
- 1/2 cup tomato, chopped
- 1/2 cup onion, chopped
- 1 1/2 tsp. curry powder
- 1/2 tsp. paprika
- 2 cups vegetable stock
- 1 tsp. olive oil
- 1/2 tsp. garlic, minced

Directions:

1. In a saucepan, add oil, garlic, and onion and sauté for 3 minutes over medium heat.
2. Add remaining ingredients into the saucepan and bring to boil.
3. Reduce heat and cover and simmer for 10 minutes.
4. Puree the soup using a blender until smooth.
5. Stir well and serve warm.

Nutrition: Calories 70; Fat 2.7 G; Carbohydrates 13.8 G; Sugar 6.3 G; Protein 1.9 G; Cholesterol 0 Mg

51. Cauliflower Spinach Soup

Preparation time: 45 minutes

Cooking time: 25 minutes

Servings: 5

Ingredients:

- 1/2 cup unsweetened coconut milk
- 5 oz. fresh spinach, chopped
- 5 watercress, chopped
- 8 cups vegetable stock
- 1 lb. cauliflower, chopped
- Salt

Directions:

1. Add stock and cauliflower in a large saucepan and bring to boil over medium heat for 15 minutes.
2. Add spinach and watercress and cook for another 10 minutes.
3. Remove from heat and puree the soup using a blender until smooth.
4. Add coconut milk and stir well. Season with salt.
5. Stir well and serve hot.

Nutrition: Calories 153; Fat 8.3 G; Carbohydrates 8.7 G; Sugar 4.3 G; Protein 11.9 G; Cholesterol 0 Mg

52. Avocado Mint Soup

Preparation time: 10 minutes

Cooking time: 10 minutes

Servings: 2

Ingredients:

- 1 medium avocado, peeled, pitted, and cut into pieces
- 1 cup coconut milk
- 2 romaine lettuce leaves
- 20 fresh mint leaves
- 1 tbsp. fresh lime juice
- 1/8 tsp. salt

Directions:

1. Add all ingredients into the blender and blend until smooth. Soup should be thick not as a puree.
2. Pour into the serving bowls and place in the refrigerator for 10 minutes.
3. Stir well and serve chilled.

Nutrition: Calories 268; Fat 25.6 G; Carbohydrates 10.2 G; Sugar 0.6 G; Protein 2.7 G; Cholesterol 0 Mg

53. Creamy Squash Soup

Preparation time: 35 minutes

Cooking time: 22 minutes

Servings: 8

Ingredients:

- 3 cups butternut squash, chopped
- 1 ½ cups unsweetened coconut milk
- 1 tbsp. coconut oil
- 1 tsp. dried onion flakes
- 1 tbsp. curry powder
- 4 cups water
- 1 garlic clove
- 1 tsp. kosher salt

Directions:

1. Add squash, coconut oil, onion flakes, curry powder, water, garlic, and salt into a large saucepan. Bring to boil over high heat.
2. Turn heat to medium and simmer for 20 minutes.
3. Puree the soup using a blender until smooth. Return soup to the saucepan and stir in coconut milk and cook for 2 minutes.
4. Stir well and serve hot.

Nutrition: Calories 146; Fat 12.6 G; Carbohydrates 9.4 G; Sugar 2.8 G; Protein 1.7 G; Cholesterol 0 Mg

Salads

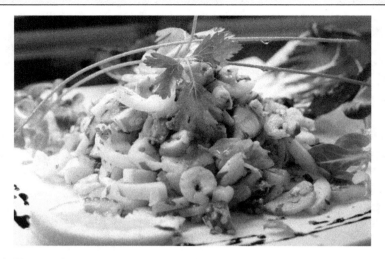

54. Romaine Lettuce and Radicchios Mix

Preparation time: 6 minutes

Cooking time: 0 minutes

Servings: 4

Ingredients:

- 2 tablespoons olive oil
- A pinch of salt and black pepper
- 2 spring onions, chopped
- 3 tablespoons Dijon mustard
- Juice of 1 lime
- ½ cup basil, chopped
- 4 cups romaine lettuce heads, chopped
- 3 radicchios, sliced

Directions:

1. In a salad bowl, mix the lettuce with the spring onions and the other ingredients, toss and serve.

Nutrition: Calories 87, Fats 2 g, Fiber 1 g, Carbs 1 g, Protein 2 g

55. Greek Salad

Preparation Time: 15 Minutes

Cooking Time: 15 Minutes

Servings: 5

Ingredients:

For Dressing:

- ½ teaspoon black pepper
- ¼ teaspoon salt
- ½ teaspoon oregano
- 1 tablespoon garlic powder
- 2 tablespoons Balsamic
- 1/3 cup olive oil

Ingredients for Salad:

- ½ cup sliced black olives
- ½ cup chopped parsley, fresh
- 1 small red onion, thin-sliced
- 1 cup cherry tomatoes, sliced
- 1 bell pepper, yellow, chunked
- 1 cucumber, peeled, quarter and slice
- 4 cups chopped romaine lettuce
- ½ teaspoon salt
- 2 tablespoons olive oil

Directions:

1. In a small bowl, blend all of the ingredients for the dressing and let this set in the refrigerator while you make the salad.

2. To assemble the salad, mix together all the ingredients in a large-sized bowl and toss the veggies gently but thoroughly to mix.

3. Serve the salad with the dressing in amounts as desired

Nutrition: Calories 234, Fat 16.1 g, Protein 5 g, Carbs 48 g

56. Asparagus And Smoked Salmon Salad

Preparation time: 15 minutes

Cooking time: 10 minutes

Servings: 8

Ingredients:

- 1 lb. fresh asparagus, trimmed and cut into 1 inch pieces
- 1/2 cup pecans, broken into pieces
- 2 heads red leaf lettuce, rinsed and torn
- 1/2 cup frozen green peas, thawed
- 1/4 lb. smoked salmon, cut into 1 inch chunks
- 1/4 cup olive oil
- 2 tbsps. lemon juice
- 1 tsp. Dijon mustard
- 1/2 tsp. salt
- 1/4 tsp. pepper

Directions:

1. Boil a pot of water. Stir in asparagus and cook for 5 minutes until tender. Let it drain; set aside.

2. In a skillet, cook the pecans over medium heat for 5 minutes, stirring constantly until lightly toasted.

3. Combine the asparagus, toasted pecans, salmon, peas, and red leaf lettuce and toss in a large bowl.

4. In another bowl, combine lemon juice, pepper, Dijon mustard, salt, and olive oil. You can coat the salad with the dressing or serve it on its side.

Nutrition: Calories: 159 calories; Total Carbohydrate: 7 g Cholesterol: 3 mg Total Fat: 12.9 g Protein: 6 g Sodium: 304 mg

57. Shrimp Cobb Salad

Preparation time: 25 minutes

Cooking time: 10 minutes

Serving: 2

Ingredients:

- 4 slices center-cut bacon
- 1 lb. large shrimp, peeled and deveined
- 1/2 tsp. ground paprika
- 1/4 tsp. ground black pepper
- 1/4 tsp. salt, divided
- 2 1/2 tbsps. Fresh lemon juice
- 1 1/2 tbsps. Extra-virgin olive oil
- 1/2 tsp. whole grain Dijon mustard
- 1 (10 oz.) package romaine lettuce hearts, chopped
- 2 cups cherry tomatoes, quartered
- 1 ripe avocado, cut into wedges
- 1 cup shredded carrots

Directions:

1. In a large skillet over medium heat, cook the bacon for 4 minutes on each side till crispy.

2. Take away from the skillet and place on paper towels; let cool for 5 minutes. Break the bacon into bits. Pour out most of the bacon fat, leaving behind only 1 tbsp. in the skillet. Bring the skillet back to medium-high heat. Add black pepper and paprika to the shrimp for seasoning. Cook the shrimp around 2

minutes each side until it is opaque. Sprinkle with 1/8 tsp. of salt for seasoning.

3.   Combine the remaining 1/8 tsp. of salt, mustard, olive oil and lemon juice together in a small bowl. Stir in the romaine hearts.

4.   On each serving plate, place on 1 and 1/2 cups of romaine lettuce. Add on top the same amounts of avocado, carrots, tomatoes, shrimp and bacon.

Nutrition: Calories: 528   calories;Total   Carbohydrate: 22.7   g Cholesterol: 365 mg Total Fat: 28.7 g Protein: 48.9 g Sodium: 1166 mg

58. Sodium: 704 mg Tomatoes and Tuna Salad

Prep: 20 minutes

Ready in: 20 minutes

Servings: 5

Ingredients:

- 1 can (12 oz.) tuna, drained and flaked
- 4 oz. cheddar cheese, cut into 1/4-inch cubes
- 1/2 to 3/4 cup mayonnaise
- 1/2 cup chopped celery
- 1/4 cup chopped onion
- 2 tbsps. chopped dill pickle
- 1 tbsp. dill pickle juice
- 1/4 tsp. salt
- 1/8 tsp. each celery seed and pepper
- 5 medium tomatoes, cored
- Bacon bits, optional

Directions:

1. Mix pepper, celery seed, salt, pickle juice, pickle, onion, celery, mayonnaise, cheese and tuna in a bowl. Keep chilled. Chop tomatoes, not quite through, into quarters; add onto separate dishes and spread apart. Scoop half cup of salad into each. Use bacon bit to decorate if you want.

Nutrition: Calories: 368 calories Total Carbohydrate: 9 g Cholesterol: 52 mg Total Fat: 26 g Fiber: 2 g Protein: 25 g

59. Avocado & Shrimp Chopped Salad

Preparation time: 15 minutes

Cooking time: 15 minutes

Serving: 4

Ingredients:

- 5 tbsps. Reduced-fat sour cream
- 3 tbsps. Grape seed oil or extra-virgin olive oil
- 3 tbsps. Cider vinegar
- 2 tbsps. Chopped fresh cilantro
- 1 tbsp. chopped fresh dill
- 1 tbsp. minced shallot
- 2 cloves garlic, minced
- ¾ tsp. dry mustard
- ¼ tsp. kosher salt
- 1 lb. raw shrimp (21-25 per lb.), peeled and deveined
- 2 tsps. Extra-virgin olive oil
- 2 tsps. Finely grated lime zest
- ¼ tsp. kosher salt
- ¼ tsp. freshly ground pepper, plus more to taste
- 2 ears corn, husked
- 4 cups chopped romaine lettuce
- ¾ cup finely chopped red cabbage
- ¾ cup diced red bell pepper
- ½ cup diced red onion
- ½ cup assorted cherry tomatoes, chopped

- ½ fennel bulb, halved again, thinly sliced

- 1 avocado, diced

- 2 slices crispy cooked bacon, diced

Directions:

1. To make the dressing: In a blender or food processor, puree the dressing ingredients until it turns smooth.

2. To make salad and shrimp: Preparation are the grill by preheating to medium or heat a grill pan on medium heat.

3. Then toss shrimp with 1/4 tsp. pepper, salt, lime zest and 2 tsps. Oil.

4. Then grill corn for 6-10 minutes, occasionally flipping, until slightly charred. Grill the shrimp for 3-5 minutes in total, turning once, until cooked through. Move the shrimp and corn to a cutting board; cut off the kernels from the cob.

5. Chop the shrimp into bite-size portions.

6. In a large bowl, mix bacon, avocado, fennel, tomatoes, onion, bell pepper, cabbage and lettuce. Then mix in the dressing, corn and shrimp; coat by tossing. Add pepper to taste.

Nutrition: Calories: 398 calories;Total Carbohydrate: 21 gCholesterol: 171 mg Total Fat: 25 g Fiber: 8 g Protein: 26 g Sodium: 374 mgSugar: 6 g Saturated Fat: 5 g

60. Tropical Style Radicchio Salad

Preparation time: 15 minutes

Cooking time: 0 minutes

Servings: 6

Ingredients:
- ½ teaspoon black pepper
- ½ teaspoon salt
- 2 tablespoons orange juice
- ¼ cup basil leaves, chopped, firmly packed
- 2 cups pineapple, fresh, finely chop
- 2 tablespoons coconut oil
- 2 medium heads radicchio, cut into quarters from top to the bottom

Directions:
1. Heat the oven to 450°f.
2. Use the coconut oil to brush both sides of the pieces of radicchio.
3. Bake the radicchio for ten minutes, turning over after five minutes. Allow the radicchio to cool. When it has cooled to room temperature, slice it very thinly, to look like chopped cabbage and then place it in a large-sized bowl.
4. Add in the pepper, salt, orange juice, basil, and pineapple and toss the ingredients gently but well to mix them together and coat all pieces well.
5. You can serve it right away or keep it in the refrigerator for no more than 1 day.

Nutrition: Calories 40, Carbs 25 g, Fat 2 g, Fiber 20 g

61. Winter Vegetable Salad

Preparation time: 10 minutes

Cooking time: 40 minutes

Servings: 3

Ingredients:

For Salad:

- 4 cups salad mixed greens, packed
- 2 tablespoons balsamic vinegar
- 1 tablespoon olive oil
- 2 tablespoons basil, dried
- 1 tablespoon coriander, dried
- 1 teaspoon rosemary
- 1 teaspoon marjoram
- 2 tablespoons parsley, fresh, chop finely
- 1 teaspoon black pepper
- ½ teaspoon salt

Ingredients for Roasted Vegetables:

- 1 tablespoon olive oil
- ½ teaspoon salt
- 1 teaspoon black pepper
- 2 parsnips
- 2 carrots
- 10 baby red potatoes
- 1 small butternut squash
- 1 red onion

Directions:

1. Heat the oven to 400°f.

2. Wash the potatoes, carrots, and parsnips and dry them with a paper towel. Wipe off the squash and the onion and peel them.

3. Chop all of the vegetables into bite-sized chunks. Place all of the chunks into a large-sized bowl with the pepper, salt, and olive oil.

4. Toss all of the vegetables in the bowl with the olive oil until they are well coated. Spread out the oiled veggies on a cookie sheet and bake them in the oven for forty minutes.

5. While the veggies are roasting, you can mix up the dressing for the salad.

6. Mix the balsamic vinegar with the olive oil and all of the pepper, salt, and herbs.

7. When you take the vegetables from the oven, divide them into servings and pour the dressing over the top of the veggie servings as personally desired.

Nutrition: Calories 483 Fat 12 g Carbs 85 g Fiber 17 g Protein 11 g

62. Asian Salmon Salad

Preparation time: 15 minutes

Cooking time: 0

Servings: 4

Ingredients:

- 1/4 cup Heinz Tomato Ketchup
- 3 tbsps. Teriyaki sauce
- 2 tbsps. Lime juice
- 2 tbsps. Sesame oil
- 2 tbsps. Brown sugar
- 8 cups lightly packed mesclun salad greens
- 2 (7.5 oz.) cans canned salmon, skin and bones removed
- 1 cup thinly sliced carrot
- 1 cup thinly sliced cucumber
- 1/4 cup sliced radish
- 1/4 cup lightly packed cilantro leaves
- 1 tsp. toasted sesame seeds

Directions:

1. Stir brown sugar, sesame oil, and lime juice and teriyaki sauce with ketchup to blend well. Reserve.

2. In a large bowl, add the salad greens. Separate large chunks of salmon. Add radish, coriander leaves, cucumber and carrot together with salmon into the bowl. Add enough dressing and gently toss till the Ingredients are coated. Season to taste with more dressing. Just before serving, sprinkle sesame seeds over.

Nutrition: Calories: 340 calories; Total Carbohydrate: 22.8 g Cholesterol: 47 mg Total Fat: 15.4 g Protein: 28.6 g Sodium: 1099 mg

63. Crab Salad Melts

Preparation time: 15 minutes

Cooking time: 25 minutes

Servings: 4

Ingredients:

- 3 asparagus spears, or 12 snow peas, trimmed and thinly sliced (about ⅓ cup)
- 8 oz. crabmeat, any shells or cartilage removed
- ⅓ cup finely chopped celery
- ¼ cup finely chopped red bell pepper
- 1 scallion, finely chopped
- 4 tsps. lemon juice
- 1 tbsp. low-fat mayonnaise
- ¼ tsp. Old Bay seasoning
- 2-5 dashes hot sauce
- Freshly ground pepper, to taste
- 4 whole-wheat English muffins, split and toasted
- ½ cup shredded Swiss cheese

Directions:

1. In the oven's upper third, set the rack and preheat the broiler.
2. In a medium microwavable bowl, arrange snow peas or asparagus and add 1 tsp of water. Microwave for 30 seconds, covered. Stir pepper, hot sauce to taste, Old Bay seasoning, mayonnaise, lemon juice, scallion, bell pepper, celery and crab till combined.
3. On a large baking sheet, arrange English muffin halves with the cut side facing up. Generously spread over each half with 1/4 cup of crab salad and sprinkle 1 tbsp. of cheese over each. Broil for 3-6 minutes to melt the cheese.

Nutrition: Calories: 258 calories; Total Carbohydrate: 30 g Cholesterol: 53 mg Total Fat: 7 g Fiber: 5 g Protein: 22 g Sodium: 539 mg Sugar: 7 g Saturated Fat: 3 g

64. Crab-stuffed Avocados

Preparation time: 20 minutes

Cooking time: 20 minutes

Servings: 2

Ingredients:

1. 1 can (6 oz.) crabmeat, drained, flaked and cartilage removed
2. 1/2 cup sliced celery
3. 1/2 cup shredded lettuce
4. 3 tbsps. mayonnaise
5. 1 tsp. finely chopped onion
6. 1/2 tsp. lemon juice
7. 1/8 to 1/4 tsp. seafood seasoning
8. 1/8 tsp. paprika
9. 1 medium ripe avocado, halved and pitted

Directions:

1. Mix the first 8 ingredients in a bowl, then scoop on avocado halves. Serve promptly.

Nutrition: Calories: 262 calories Total Carbohydrate: 11 g Cholesterol: 78 mg Total Fat: 17 g Fiber: 5 g Protein: 20 g Sodium: 543 mg

65. Tomato Salad

Preparation time: 15 minutes

Cooking time: 0 minutes

Servings: 6

Ingredients:

- ¼ cup basil leaves, chopped fresh
- 1 cup yellow tomatoes, sliced thinly
- 1 cup red tomatoes, sliced thinly
- 2 tablespoons chives, chop finely
- 1-pint grape tomatoes, halved
- 1 teaspoon black pepper
- ½ teaspoon salt
- 2 tablespoons balsamic vinegar
- ¼ cup olive oil

Directions:

1. Mix together in a medium-sized bowl the salt, pepper, balsamic vinegar, and the olive oil until well blended.
2. Put the tomatoes in this mix and toss them gently to coat them well.
3. Sprinkle the top of the mix with the chives and the fresh basil.

Nutrition: Calories 105, Fat 9.5g, Protein 1g, Carbs 6g

66. Cauliflower Sweet Potato Salad

Preparation time: 20 minutes

Cooking time: 30 minutes

Servings: 8

Ingredients:

- ½ cup cranberries, dried
- 8 cups lettuce, any variety, torn
- 1 tablespoon balsamic vinegar
- 1 teaspoon black pepper
- 1 teaspoon salt
- 7 tablespoons olive oil, divided
- 1 small head cauliflower, broken into florets
- 1 ½ pound sweet potatoes, cut into ½ inch wide wedges

Directions:

1. Heat the oven to 425°f. Mix together in a medium-sized bowl the cauliflower florets and the sweet potato wedges with the pepper, salt, and tablespoons of the olive oil. Spread these out on a cookie sheet and bake them for thirty minutes and then let them cool slightly.

2. During the time that the veggies are roasting, mix together the balsamic vinegar and the remainder of the olive oil in a large bowl.

3. Then add in the dried cranberries, lettuce, and the cooled roasted veggies.

4. Toss this mixture well to coat all pieces and serve immediately.

Nutrition: Calories 150, Fat 12 g, Carbs 11 g, Fiber 3 g, Protein 5 g

67. Winter Vegetable Salad

Preparation time: 10 minutes

Cooking time: 40 minutes

Servings: 3

Ingredients:

For Salad:

- 4 cups salad mixed greens, packed
- 2 tablespoons balsamic vinegar
- 1 tablespoon olive oil
- 2 tablespoons basil, dried
- 1 tablespoon coriander, dried
- 1 teaspoon rosemary
- 1 teaspoon marjoram
- 2 tablespoons parsley, fresh, chop finely
- 1 teaspoon black pepper
- ½ teaspoon salt

Ingredients for Roasted Vegetables:

- 1 tablespoon olive oil
- ½ teaspoon salt
- 1 teaspoon black pepper
- 2 parsnips
- 2 carrots
- 10 baby red potatoes
- 1 small butternut squash
- 1 red onion

Directions:

1. Heat the oven to 400°f.

2. Wash the potatoes, carrots, and parsnips and dry them with a paper towel. Wipe off the squash and the onion and peel them.

3. Chop all of the vegetables into bite-sized chunks. Place all of the chunks into a large-sized bowl with the pepper, salt, and olive oil.

4. Toss all of the vegetables in the bowl with the olive oil until they are well coated. Spread out the oiled veggies on a cookie sheet and bake them in the oven for forty minutes.

5. While the veggies are roasting, you can mix up the dressing for the salad.

6. Mix the balsamic vinegar with the olive oil and all of the pepper, salt, and herbs.

7. When you take the vegetables from the oven, divide them into servings and pour the dressing over the top of the veggie servings as personally desired.

Nutrition: Calories 483 Fat 12 g Carbs 85 g Fiber 17 g Protein 11 g

Pescatarian Snacks

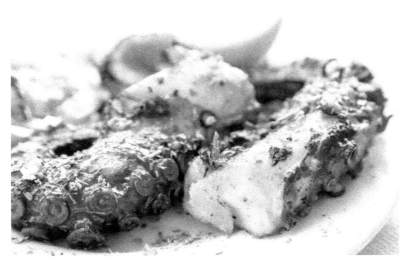

68. Grilled Salmon Burger

Preparation Time: 15 minutes

Cooking time: 10 minutes

Servings: 4

Ingredients:

- 16 ounces (450 g) pink salmon fillet, minced

- 1 cup (250 g) prepared mashed potatoes

- 1 shallot (about 40 g), chopped

- 1 large egg (about 60 g), lightly beaten

- 2 tablespoons (7 g) fresh coriander, chopped

- 4 Hamburger buns (about 60 g each), split

- 1 large tomato (about 150 g), sliced

- 8 (15 g) Romaine lettuce leaves

- 1/4 cup (60 g) mayonnaise

- Salt and freshly ground black pepper
- Cooking oil spray

Directions:

1. Combine the salmon, mashed potatoes, shallot, egg, and coriander in a mixing bowl. Season with salt and pepper.
2. Spoon about 2 tablespoons of mixture and form into patties.
3. Preheat your grill or griddle on high. Grease with cooking oil spray.
4. Grill the salmon patties for 4-5 minutes on each side or until cooked through. Transfer to a clean plate and cover to keep warm.
5. Spread some mayonnaise on the bottom half of buns. Top with lettuce, salmon patty, and tomato. Cover with bun tops.
6. Serve and enjoy.

Nutrition: Energy - 395 calories Fat - 18.0 g Carbohydrates - 38.8 g Protein - 21.8 g Sodium - 383 mg

Easy Salmon Burger

Preparation Time: 15 minutes

Cooking time: 15 minutes

Servings: 6

Ingredients:

- 16 ounces (450 g) pink salmon, minced
- 1 cup (250 g) prepared mashed potatoes
- 1 medium (110 g) onion, chopped
- 1 stalk celery (about 60 g), finely chopped
- 1 large egg (about 60 g), lightly beaten
- 2 tablespoons (7 g) fresh cilantro, chopped
- 1 cup (100 g) breadcrumbs
- Vegetable oil, for deep frying
- Salt and freshly ground black pepper

Directions:

1. Combine the salmon, mashed potatoes, onion, celery, egg, and cilantro in a mixing bowl. Season to taste and mix thoroughly. Spoon about 2 Tbsp. mixture, roll in breadcrumbs, and then form into small patties.
2. Heat oil in non-stick frying pan. Cook your salmon patties for 5 minutes on each side or until golden brown and crispy.
3. Serve in burger buns and with coleslaw on the side if desired.
4. Enjoy.

Nutrition: Energy - 230 calories Fat - 7.9 g Carbs - 20.9 g Protein - 18.9 g Sodium - 298 mg

69. Salmon Sandwich with Avocado and Egg

Preparation Time: 15 minutes

Cooking time: 10 minutes

Servings: 4

Ingredients:

- 8 ounces (250 g) smoked salmon, thinly sliced
- 1 medium (200 g) ripe avocado, thinly sliced
- 4 large poached eggs (about 60 g each)
- 4 slices whole wheat bread (about 30 g each)
- 2 cups (60 g) arugula or baby rocket
- Salt and freshly ground black pepper

Directions:

1. Place 1 bread slice on a plate top with arugula, avocado, salmon, and poached egg. Season with salt and pepper. Repeat procedure for the remaining ingredients.
2. Serve and enjoy.

Nutrition: Energy - 310 calories Fat - 18.2 g Carbohydrates - 16.4 g Protein - 21.3 g Sodium - 383 mg

70. Salmon Spinach and Cottage Cheese Sandwich

Preparation Time: 15 minutes

Cooking time: 10 minutes

Servings: 4

Ingredients:

- 4 ounces (125 g) cottage cheese
- 1/4 cup (15 g) chives, chopped
- 1 teaspoon (5 g) capers
- 1/2 teaspoon (2.5 g) grated lemon rind
- 4 (2 oz. or 60 g) smoked salmon
- 2 cups (60 g) loose baby spinach
- 1 medium (110 g) red onion, sliced thinly
- 8 slices rye bread (about 30 g each)
- Kosher salt and freshly ground black pepper

Directions:

1. Preheat your griddle or Panini press.
2. Mix together cottage cheese, chives, capers, and lemon rind in a small bowl.
3. Spread and divide the cheese mixture on 4 bread slices. Top with spinach, onion slices, and smoked salmon.
4. Cover with remaining bread slices.
5. Grill the sandwiches until golden and grill marks form on both sides.
6. Transfer to a serving dish.
7. Serve and enjoy.

Nutrition: Energy - 261 calories Fat 9.9 g Carbohydrates 22.9 g Protein 19.9 g Sodium - 1226 mg

71. Salmon Feta and Pesto Wrap

Preparation Time: 15 minutes

Cooking time: 10 minutes

Servings: 4

Ingredients:

- 8 ounces (250 g) smoked salmon fillet, thinly sliced
- 1 cup (150 g) feta cheese
- 8 (15 g) Romaine lettuce leaves
- 4 (6-inch) pita bread
- 1/4 cup (60 g) basil pesto sauce

Directions:

1. Place 1 pita bread on a plate. Top with lettuce, salmon, feta cheese, and pesto sauce. Fold or roll to enclose filling. Repeat procedure for the remaining ingredients.
2. Serve and enjoy.

Nutrition: Energy 379 calories Fat 17.7 g Carbohydrates 36.6 g Protein - 18.4 g Sodium - 554 mg

72. Salmon Cream Cheese and Onion on Bagel

Preparation Time: 15 minutes

Cooking time: 10 minutes

Servings: 4

Ingredients:

- 8 ounces (250 g) smoked salmon fillet, thinly sliced
- 1/2 cup (125 g) cream cheese
- 1 medium (110 g) onion, thinly sliced
- 4 bagels (about 80g each), split
- 2 tablespoons (7 g) fresh parsley, chopped
- Freshly ground black pepper, to taste

Directions:

1. Spread the cream cheese on each bottom's half of bagels. Top with salmon and onion, season with pepper, sprinkle with parsley and then cover with bagel tops.
2. Serve and enjoy.

Nutrition: Energy 309 calories Fat 14.1 g Carbohydrates 32.0 g Protein 14.7 g Sodium 571 mg

73. Greek Baklava

Preparation time: 20 minutes

Cooking time: 20 minutes

Servings: 18

Ingredients:

- 1 (16 oz.) package phyllo dough
- 1 lb. chopped nuts
- 1 cup butter
- 1 tsp. ground cinnamon
- 1 cup water
- 1 cup white sugar
- 1 tsp. vanilla extract
- 1/2 cup honey

Directions:

1. Preheat the oven to 175°C or 350°Fahrenheit. Spread butter on the sides and bottom of a 9-in by 13-in pan.

2. Chop the nuts then mix with cinnamon; set it aside. Unfurl the phyllo dough then halve the whole stack to fit the pan. Use a damp cloth to cover the phyllo to prevent drying as you proceed. Put two phyllo sheets in the pan then butter well. Repeat to make eight layered phyllo sheets. Scatter 2-3 tbsps. nut mixture over the sheets then place two more phyllo sheets on top, butter then sprinkle with nuts. Layer as you go. The final layer should be six to eight phyllo sheets deep.

3. Make square or diamond shapes with a sharp knife up to the bottom of pan. You can slice into four long rows for diagonal shapes. Bake until crisp and golden for 50 minutes.

4. Meanwhile, boil water and sugar until the sugar melts to make the sauce; mix in honey and vanilla. Let it simmer for 20 minutes.

5. Take the baklava out of the oven then drizzle with sauce right away; cool. Serve the baklava in cupcake papers. You can also freeze them without cover. The baklava will turn soggy when wrapped.

Nutrition: Calories: 393 calories; Total Carbohydrate: 37.5 g Cholesterol: 27 mg Total Fat: 25.9 g Protein: 6.1 g Sodium: 196 mg

74. Glazed Bananas in Phyllo Nut Cups

Preparation time: 30 minutes

Cooking time: 45 minutes

Servings: 6 servings. |

Ingredients:

- 3/4 cup shelled pistachios

- 1/2 cup sugar

- 1 tsp. ground cinnamon

- 4 sheets phyllo dough, (14 inches x 9 inches)

- 1/4 cup butter, melted

- SAUCE:

- 3/4 cup butter, cubed

- 3/4 cup packed brown sugar

- 3 medium firm bananas, sliced

- 1/4 tsp. ground cinnamon

- 3 to 4 cups vanilla ice cream

Directions:

1. Finely chop sugar and pistachios in a food processor; move to a bowl then mix in cinnamon. Slice each phyllo sheet to 6 four-inch squares, get rid of the trimmings. Pile the squares then use plastic wrap to cover.

2. Slather melted butter on each square one at a time then scatter a heaping tablespoonful of pistachio mixture. Pile 3 squares, flip each at an angle to misalign the corners. Force each stack

on the sides and bottom of an oiled eight-oz. custard cup. Bake for 15-20 minutes in a 350 degrees F oven until golden; cool for 5 minutes. Move to a wire rack to completely cool.

3. Melt and boil brown sugar and butter in a saucepan to make the sauce; lower heat. Mix in cinnamon and bananas gently; heat completely. Put ice cream in the phyllo cups until full then put banana sauce on top. Serve right away.

Nutrition: Calories: 735 calories Total Carbohydrate: 82 g Cholesterol: 111 mg Total Fat: 45 g Fiber: 3 g Protein: 7 g Sodium: 468 mg

75. Salmon Apple Salad Sandwich

Preparation Time: 15 minutes

Cooking Time: 10 minutes

Servings: 4

Ingredients:

- 4 ounces (125 g) canned pink salmon, drained and flaked
- 1 medium (180 g) red apple, cored and diced
- 1 celery stalk (about 60 g), chopped
- 1 shallot (about 40 g), finely chopped
- 1/3 cup (85 g) light mayonnaise
- 8 slices whole grain bread (about 30 g each), toasted
- 8 (15 g) Romaine lettuce leaves
- Salt and freshly ground black pepper

Directions:

1. Combine the salmon, apple, celery, shallot, and mayonnaise in a mixing bowl. Season with salt and pepper.
2. Place 1 slices bread on a plate, top with lettuce and salmon salad, and then covers with another slice of bread. Repeat procedure for the remaining ingredients.
3. Serve and enjoy.

Nutrition: Energy - 305 calories Fat - 11.3 g Carbohydrates - 40.4 g Protein - 15.1 g Sodium - 469 mg

76. Smoked Salmon and Cheese on Rye Bread

Preparation Time: 15 minutes

Cooking time: 10 minutes

Servings: 4

Ingredients:

- 8 ounces (250 g) smoked salmon, thinly sliced

- 1/3 cup (85 g) mayonnaise

- 2 tablespoons (30 ml) lemon juice

- 1 tablespoon (15 g) Dijon mustard

- 1 teaspoon (3 g) garlic, minced

- 4 slices cheddar cheese (about 2 oz. or 30 g each)

- 8 slices rye bread (about 2 oz. or 30 g each)

- 8 (15 g) Romaine lettuce leaves

- Salt and freshly ground black pepper

Directions:

1. Mix together the mayonnaise, lemon juice, mustard, and garlic in a small bowl. Flavor with salt and pepper and set aside.

2. Spread dressing on 4 bread slices. Top with lettuce, salmon, and cheese. Cover with remaining rye bread slices.

3. Serve and enjoy.

Nutrition: Energy - 365 calories Fat - 16.6 g Carbohydrates - 31.6 g Protein - 18.8 g Sodium - 951 mg

77. Cajun-Style Fish

Preparation time: 15 minutes

Cooking time: 25 minutes

Servings: 4

Ingredients:

- 1 cup chopped onion
- 1 clove garlic, minced
- 2 teaspoons margarine
- 1 can (15 ½ ounces) diced tomatoes, un-drained
- 1 large green bell pepper, chopped
- 2 cups cubed zucchini and/or yellow squash
- ½ teaspoon dried basil leaves
- ½ teaspoon dried thyme leaves
- ¼ teaspoon dried marjoram leaves
- 2-3 drops hot pepper sauce
- Salt and pepper, to taste
- Vegetable cooking spray
- 1 pound skinless fish fillets (flounder, sole, halibut, turbot, or other lean white fish)
- 3 cups cooked rice, warm

Directions:

1. Sauté onion and garlic in margarine in large skillet until almost tender, about 5 minutes. Add tomatoes, green pepper, squash, and herbs. Heat to boiling; reduce heat and cook, covered,

about 10 minutes or until vegetables are tender. Season to taste with hot pepper sauce, salt, and pepper.

2. While vegetables are cooking, cook fish. Spray large skillet with cooking spray; heat over medium heat until hot. Add fish and cook over medium heat until hot. Add fish and cook over medium heat until fish is tender and flakes with a fork, about 4 minutes on each side. Season to taste with salt and pepper. Spoon rice onto large serving platter; top with vegetables and fish.

3. Enjoy!

Nutrition: Calories: 221 % Calories from fat: 10 Fat (gm): 2.6 Sat. fat (gm): 0.4 Cholesterol (mg): 35.5 Sodium (mg): 193 Protein (gm): 16.5 Carbohydrate (gm): 32.7

78. Pan-Fried Trout

Preparation time: 15 minutes

Cooking time: 10 minutes

Servings: 4

Ingredients:

- 1 ¼ pounds trout fillets
- 1/3 cup white, or yellow, cornmeal
- ¼ teaspoon anise seeds
- ¼ teaspoon black pepper
- ½ cup minced cilantro, or parsley
- Vegetable cooking spray
- Lemon wedges

Directions:

1. Coat fish with combined cornmeal, spices, and cilantro, pressing it gently into fish.Spray large skillet with cooking spray; heat over medium heat until hot. Add fish and cook until fish is tender and flakes with fork, about 5 minutes on each side. Serve with lemon wedges.

2. Enjoy!

Nutrition: Calories: 207 % Calories from fat: 23 Fat (gm): 5.2 Sat. fat (gm): 1 Cholesterol (mg): 81.1 Sodium (mg): 42 Protein (gm): 30.2 Carbohydrate (gm): 8

79. Sole with Rosemary Potatoes

Preparation time: 15 minutes

Cooking time: 1 hour

Servings: 4

Ingredients:

- 4 small baking potatoes, cut into wedges
- Vegetable cooking spray
- 2 tablespoons dried rosemary leaves
- ½ teaspoon garlic powder
- ¼ teaspoon pepper
- 4 shallots, minced
- 1 small red onion, chopped
- 1 large clove garlic, minced
- 1 ¼ pounds sole fillets

Directions:

1. Place potatoes on baking sheet; spray lightly with cooking spray and sprinkle with rosemary, garlic powder, and pepper. Bake potatoes at 400 degrees until fork-tender, about 45 minutes. About 15 minutes before potatoes are done, spray large skillet with cooking spray; heat over medium heat until hot. Sauté shallots, onion, and garlic until tender, about 5 minutes. Fold each sole fillet in half and add to skillet. Cook fish over medium heat until fish is tender and flakes with a fork, about 6 minutes, turning once. Place fish on serving platter; spoon shallot mixture over fish. Surround with hot rosemary potatoes.
2. Enjoy!

Nutrition: Calories: 279 % Calories from fat: 7 Fat (gm): 2.1 Sat. fat (gm): 0.6 Cholesterol (mg): 68 Sodium (mg): 127 Protein (gm): 30.1 Carbohydrate (gm): 34.4

80. Sardines on Crackers

Preparation time: 5 minutes

Cooking time: 0

Servings: 4

Ingredients:

- 4 whole-grain Scandinavian-style crackers, such as Wasa, Ry Krisp, Ryvita, Kavli

- 8-12 canned sardines, preferably packed in olive oil

- 4 lemon wedges

Directions:

1. Place 2 to 3 sardines on top of each cracker. Complete with a squeeze of lemon.

Nutrition: Calories: 64 calories; Total Carbohydrate: 8 g Cholesterol: 20 mg Total Fat: 2 g Fiber: 1 g Protein: 4 g Sodium: 66 mg Sugar: 1 g Saturated Fat: 0 g

81. Sardines and Pineapple Sandwich Toast

Preparation time: 10 minutes

Cooking time: 15 minutes

Servings: 2

Ingredients:

- 4 slices bread
- 1 tbsp. mayonnaise
- 1 pinch salt and ground black pepper
- 2 tsps. marmalade
- 4 potato chips, crushed
- 2 pieces pineapple, thinly sliced
- 4 sardines, drained, or to taste

Directions:

1. Preheat your sandwich maker following the manufacturer's directions.
2. Spread 2 slices of bread with mayonnaise. Coat with marmalade. Scatter potato chips over marmalade. Layer the pineapple over chips.
3. Crumble sardines in a bowl with a fork. Scatter over the top of the pineapple slices. Flavor with pepper and salt; cover with leftover 2 slices of bread.
4. Toast in the prepared sandwich maker until crispy and brown, about 5 minutes.

Nutrition: Calories: 271 calories; Total Carbohydrate: 33.3 g Cholesterol: 37 mg Total Fat: 10.8 g Protein: 10.1 g Sodium: 595 mg

82. Sardines With Ginger

Preparation time: 10 minutes

Cooking time: 16 minutes

Servings: 2

Ingredients

- 1 tsp. sesame oil
- 4 fresh sardines
- 3 tbsps. sake
- 2 spring onions, finely chopped
- 1 1/2 tbsps. soy sauce
- 1 1/2 tbsps. mirin (Japanese sweet rice wine)
- 2 tsps. chopped ginger

Direction

1. Heat oil over high heat in a skillet. Put in sardines and cook until golden, turning occasionally, about 3 minutes on each side. Remove onto a serving plate.

2. In a small bowl, stir chopped ginger, mirin, soy sauce, spring onions, and sake together to make sauce. Transfer the sauce over sardines to serve.

Nutrition Information Calories: 451 Kcal; Total Carbohydrate: 7 g Cholesterol: 0 mg Total Fat: 25.9 g Protein: 33.9 g Sodium: 679 mg

83. Sardines with Grilled Bread And Tomato

Preparation time

Cooking time:

Servings: 4 Servings

Ingredients:

- 2 tbsps. olive oil, plus more
- 4 (3/4"-thick) slices sourdough or country-style bread
- 12 whole fresh sardines (1–1 1/2 lbs. total), scaled, gutted, large pin bones removed
- Kosher salt, freshly ground pepper
- freshly ground pepper
- 1 large tomato, preferably heirloom, sliced
- Torn basil leaves (for serving)

Directions:

1. Preparation: Set the grill to medium-high heat; grease the grate. Brush 2 tbsps. of oil total on both sides of bread and grill, flipping from time to time, for about 4 minutes until toasted and lightly charred. Place the grilled bread to a plate.

2. Season the outside and inside of sardines with pepper and salt (no need to grease them, as their skin has so much natural oil). Grill, flipping from time to time, for 5 to 7 minutes until cooked through and lightly charred.

3. Serve sardines with tomato and grilled bread sprinkled with oil and topped with basil.

Nutrition: Calories: 486 Total Carbohydrate: 74 g Cholesterol: 18 mg Total Fat: 12 g Fiber: 4 g Protein: 21 g Sodium: 870 mg

Pescatarian Side Dishes

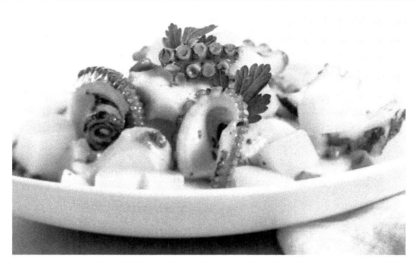

84. Creamed Coconut Curry Spinach

Preparation Time: 30 minutes

Cooking time: 30 seconds

Servings: 6

Ingredients:

- 1-pound frozen spinach, thawed and drained of moisture

- 1 small can whole fat coconut milk

- 2 tsp. yellow curry paste

- 1 tsp. lemon zest

- Cashews for garnish

Directions:

1. Heat a medium sized pan to medium high heat, then add the curry paste and cook for 30 seconds. Add a small amount of

the coconut milk and stir to combine, and then cook until the paste is aromatic.

2. Add the spinach, and then season. Separate the rest of the ingredients, from the cashews, and allow the sauce to reduce slightly.

3. Keep the sauce creamy but reduce it to coat the spinach well. Serve with chopped cashews.

Nutrition: Net carbs: 3g, Protein: 4g, Fat: 18g, Calories: 191kcal.

85. Shrimp Salad Cocktails

Preparation time: 35 minutes

Cooking time: 35 minutes

Servings: 8 servings

Ingredients:

- 2 cups mayonnaise
- 1/4 cup ketchup
- 1/4 cup lemon juice
- 1 tbsp. Worcestershire sauce
- 2 lbs. peeled and deveined cooked large shrimp
- 2 celery ribs, finely chopped
- 3 tbsps. minced fresh tarragon or 3 tsps. dried tarragon
- 1/4 tsp. salt
- 1/4 tsp. pepper
- 2 cups shredded romaine
- 2 cups seedless red and/or green grapes, halved
- 6 plum tomatoes, seeded and finely chopped
- 1/2 cup chopped peeled mango or papaya
- Minced chives or parsley

Directions:

1. Combine Worcestershire sauce, lemon juice, ketchup and mayonnaise together in a small bowl. Combine pepper, salt, tarragon, celery and shrimp together in a large bowl. Put in 1 cup of dressing toss well to coat.

2. Scoop 1 tbsp. of the dressing into 8 cocktail glasses. Layer each glass with 1/4 cup of lettuce, followed by 1/2 cup of the shrimp mixture, 1/4 cup of grapes, 1/3 cup of tomatoes and finally 1 tbsp. of mango. Spread the remaining dressing over top; sprinkle chives on top. Serve immediately.

Nutrition: Calories: 580 calories Total Carbohydrate: 16 g Cholesterol: 192 mg Total Fat: 46 g Fiber: 2 g Protein: 24 g Sodium: 670 mg

86. Garlic Chive Cauliflower Mash

Preparation Time: 20 minutes

Cooking time: 18 minutes

Servings: 5

Ingredients:

- 4 cups cauliflower
- 1/3 cup vegetarian mayonnaise
- 1 garlic clove
- 1/2 tsp. kosher salt
- 1 tbsp. water
- 1/8 tsp. pepper
- 1/4 tsp. lemon juice
- 1/2 tsp. lemon zest
- 1 tbsps. Chives, minced

Directions:

1. In a bowl that is save to microwave, add the cauliflower, mayo, garlic, water, and salt/pepper and mix until the cauliflower is well coated. Cook on high for 15-18 minutes, until the cauliflower is almost mushy.

2. Blend the mixture in a strong blender until completely smooth, adding a little more water if the mixture is too chunky. Season with the remaining ingredients and serve.

Nutrition: Net carbs: 3g, Protein: 2g, Fat: 18g, Calories: 178kcal.

87. Beet Greens With Pine Nuts Goat Cheese

Preparation Time: 25 minutes

Cooking time: 15 minutes

Servings: 3

Ingredients:

- 4 cups beet tops, washed and chopped roughly
- 1 tsp. EVOO
- 1 tbsp. no sugar added balsamic vinegar
- 2 oz. crumbled dry goat cheese
- 2 tbsps. Toasted pine nuts

Directions:

1. Warm the oil in a large pan, then cook the beet greens on medium high heat until they release their moisture. Let it cook until almost tender. Flavor with salt and pepper and remove from heat.
2. Toss the greens in a mixture of balsamic vinegar and olive oil, then top with the nuts and cheese. Serve warm.

Nutrition: Net carbs: 3.5g, Protein: 10g, Fat: 18g, Calories: 215kcal.

88. Shrimp with Dipping Sauce

Preparation time: 5 minutes

Cooking time: 15 minutes

Serving: 6

Ingredients:

- 1 tbsp. reduced-sodium soy sauce
- 2 tsps. Hot pepper sauce
- 1 tsp. canola oil
- 1/4 tsp. garlic powder
- 1/8 to 1/4 tsp. cayenne pepper
- 1 lb. uncooked medium shrimp, peeled and deveined
- 2 tbsps. Chopped green onions

Dipping Sauce:

- 3 tbsps. Reduced-sodium soy sauce
- 1 tbsp. rice vinegar
- 1 tbsp. orange juice
- 2 tsps. Sesame oil
- 2 tsps. Honey
- 1 garlic clove, minced
- 1-1/2 tsps. Minced fresh gingerroot

Directions:

1. Heat the initial 5 ingredients in a big nonstick frying pan for 30 seconds, then mix continuously. Add onions and shrimp and stir fry for 4-5 minutes or until the shrimp turns pink. Mix together the sauce ingredients and serve it with the shrimp.

Nutrition: Calories: 97 calories Total Carbohydrate: 4 g Cholesterol: 112 mg Total Fat: 3 g Fiber: 0 g Protein: 13 g Sodium: 588 mg

89. Celeriac Cauliflower Mash

Preparation Time: 20 minutes

Cooking time: 12 minutes

Servings: 6

Ingredients:

- 1 head cauliflower
- 1 small celery root
- 1/4 cup butter
- 1 tbsp. chopped rosemary
- 1 tbsp. chopped thyme
- 1 cup cream cheese

Directions:

1. Skin the celery root and cut into small pieces. Cut the cauliflower into similar sized pieces and combine.

2. Toast the herbs in the butter in a large pan, until they become fragrant. Add the cauliflower and celery root and stir to combine. Season and cook at medium high until whatever moisture is in the vegetables releases itself, then covers and cook on low for 10-12 minutes.

3. Once the vegetables are soft, remove from the heat and place them in the blender. Make it smooth, then put the cream cheese and puree again. Season and serve.

Nutrition: Net carbs: 7.3g, Protein: 5.6g, Fat: 20.8g, Calories: 225kcal.

90. Cheddar Drop Biscuits

Preparation Time: 30 minutes

Cooking time: 15 minutes

Servings: 8

Ingredients:

- 1/4 cup coconut oil
- 4 eggs
- 2 tsp. apple cider vinegar
- 1 1/2 cup coarse almond meal
- 1/2 tsp. baking powder, gluten free
- 1/2 tsp. onion powder
- 1/4 tsp. salt
- 3/4 cup cheddar cheese
- 2 tbsps. Chopped jalapenos

Directions:

1. Line a sheet tray with parchment paper, and then preheat the oven to 400F

2. Mix the wet ingredients in a bowl until combined, then reserve. Mix the dry ingredients in a separate bowl until combined, and then add them to the wet ingredients, stirring until incorporated. Fold in the cheddar cheese and jalapenos.

3. Drop the dough onto the parchment paper into eight roughly equal pieces, and then shape as desired once they are on the tray.

4. Bake until golden brown, 12-15 minutes. Rotate the tray halfway through baking so browning is even.

5. Cool slightly and serve.

Nutrition: Net carbs: 6.9g, Protein: 3.2g, Fat: 22.1g, Calories: 260kcal.

91. Roasted Radish with Fresh Herbs

Preparation Time: 15 minutes

Cooking time: 10 minutes

Servings: 4

Ingredients:

- 1 tbsp. coconut oil
- 1 bunch radishes
- 2 tbsps. Minced chives
- 1 tbsp. minced rosemary
- 1 tbsp. minced thyme

Directions:

1. Wash the radishes, and then remove the tops and stems. Cut them into quarters and reserve.

2. Add the oil to a cast iron pan, then heat to medium. Add the radishes, and then season with salt and pepper. Cook on medium heat for 6-8 minutes, until almost tender, then add the herbs and cook through.

3. The radishes can be served warm with meats or chilled with salads.

Nutrition: Net carbs: 1.8g, Protein: .9g, Fat: 13g, Calories: 133kcal.

92. Summer Bruschetta

Preparation Time: 15 min

Cooking Time: 3 hours

Servings: 4

Ingredients:

- Basil leaves (chopped) – 6
- Artichoke hearts (quartered) – ½ cup
- Kalamata olives (halved) – ¼ cup
- Capers – ¼ cup
- Roma tomatoes (diced) – 4
- Balsamic vinegar – 3 tablespoon
- Avocado oil – 3 tablespoon
- Onion powder – ¾ teaspoon
- Sea salt – ¾ teaspoon
- Black pepper – ½ teaspoon
- Garlic (minced) – 2 tablespoon

Directions:

1. Combine all the ingredients in the slow cooker and stir mix.
2. Cook for 3 hours on high, stirring the mix after every hour.

Nutrition: 152 Cal, 13g total fat, 7.5 g net carb. 1 g protein.

93. Tomato Cheddar Fondue

Preparation time: 20 minutes

Cooking time: 30 minutes

Serving: 3-1/2 cups

Ingredients:

- 1 garlic clove, halved
- 6 medium tomatoes, seeded and diced
- 2/3 cup dry white wine
- 6 tbsps. butter, cubed
- 1-1/2 tsps. dried basil
- Dash cayenne pepper
- 2 cups shredded cheddar cheese
- 1 tbsp. all-purpose flour
- Cubed French bread and cooked shrimp

Directions:

1. Rub the bottom and sides of a fondue pot with a garlic clove. Set aside and discard the garlic.

2. Combine wine, butter, basil, cayenne and tomatoes in a large saucepan. On a medium low heat, bring mixture to a simmer, then decrease heat to low. Mix cheese with flour. Add to tomato mixture gradually while stirring after each addition until cheese is melted.

3. Pour into the Preparation timeared fondue pot and keep warm. Enjoy with shrimp and bread cubes.

Nutrition: Calories: 118 calories Total Carbohydrate: 4 g Cholesterol: 30 mg Total Fat: 10 g Fiber: 1 g Protein: 4 g Sodium: 135 mg

94. Swiss Seafood Canapés

Preparation time: 20 minutes

Cooking time: 25 minutes

Servings: 4 dozen.

Ingredients:

- 1 can (6 oz.) small shrimp, rinsed and drained
- 1 package (6 oz.) frozen crabmeat, thawed
- 1 cup shredded Swiss cheese
- 2 hard-boiled large eggs, chopped
- 1/4 cup finely chopped celery
- 1/4 cup mayonnaise
- 1/4 cup French salad dressing or seafood cocktail sauce
- 2 green onions, chopped
- Dash salt
- 1 loaf (16 oz.) snack rye bread

Directions:

1. Mix the first nine ingredients in a large bowl. Put bread on ungreased baking sheets. Broil for 1 to 2 minutes, 4 to 6-inches from the heat or until lightly browned. Flip slices over; spread 1 rounded tablespoonful of seafood mixture on each. Broil for 4 to 5 more minutes or until heated through.

Nutrition: Calories: 57 calories Total Carbohydrate: 5 g Cholesterol: 22 mg Total Fat: 3 g Fiber: 1 g Protein: 3 g Sodium: 143 mg

95. Squash & Zucchini

Preparation Time: 5 min

Cooking Time: 4-6 hours

Servings: 6

Ingredients:

- Zucchini (sliced and quartered) – 2 cups
- Yellow squash (sliced and quartered) – 2 cups
- Pepper – ¼ teaspoon
- Italian seasoning – 1 teaspoon
- Garlic powder – 1 teaspoon
- Sea salt – ½ teaspoon
- Butter (cubed) – ¼ cup
- Parmesan cheese (grated) – ¼ cup

Directions:

1. Combine all the ingredients in the slow cooker.
2. Cook covered for 4-6 hours on low.

Nutrition: 122 Cal, 9.9 g fat, 369 mg sodium, 5.4 g carb. 1.7 g fiber, 4.2 g protein

96. Tasty Shrimp Spread

Preparation time: 15 minutes

Cooking time: 20 minutes

Serving: 2-1/2 cups

Ingredients:

- 1 package (8 oz.) cream cheese, softened
- 1/4 cup butter, softened
- 1/4 cup mayonnaise
- 1/2 lb. peeled and deveined cooked shrimp, finely chopped
- 1 medium onion, chopped
- Assorted crackers and/or fresh vegetables

Directions:

1. Combine mayonnaise, butter and cream cheese together in a small bowl. Mix in onion and shrimp. Refrigerate with a cover till serving. Serve with crackers and/or vegetables if you want.

Nutrition: Calories: 189 calories Total Carbohydrate: 2 g Cholesterol: 73 mg Total Fat: 17 g Fiber: 0 g Protein: 7 g Sodium: 163 mg

97. Creamy Coconut Spinach

Preparation Time: 10 min

Cooking Time: 25 min

Servings: 2

Ingredients:

- Baby spinach – 4 cups
- Coconut milk – ¼ cup
- Nutmeg – 1/8 teaspoon
- Granulated sugar substitute – 2 teaspoon
- Cayenne pepper - 1/8 teaspoon
- Salt – to taste

Directions:

1. Heat a saucepan and warm the coconut milk in it for 2 minutes.
2. Mix in the spinach, cooking until bright green and wilted.
3. Mix in the rest of the ingredients.

Nutrition: 73 Cal, 7 g total fat, 3 g carb. 2 g fiber, 2 g protein.

Pescatarian Dessert

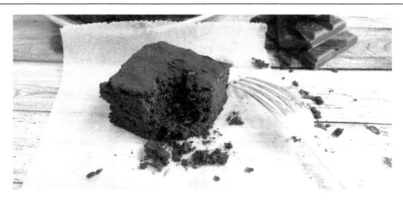

98. Ice Cream with Avocado

Preparation time: 10 minutes

Cooking time: 30 minutes

Servings: 6

Ingredients:

- 1 peeled and pitted the avocado
- 1½ tsp. of vanilla paste
- 1 c.cm. of coconut milk
- 2 tbsps. of almond butter
- Drops of stevia
- ¼ tsp. of Ceylon cinnamon

Directions:

1. Combine all ingredients in a food blender.
2. Blend until smooth.
3. Transfer the mixture into Popsicle molds and insert popsicle sticks.
4. Freeze for 4 hours or until firm and then serve.

Nutrition: Calories: 41 kcal Fats: 10 g Net Carbs 0.1 g Protein 0 g

99. Delicious Brownies

Preparation time: 10 minutes

Cooking time: 25 minutes

Servings: 4

Ingredients:

- 5 ounces of chocolate 86% (sugarless); melted
- 4 tablespoons of ghee, melted
- 3 eggs
- ½ cup of Swerve
- ¼ cup of mascarpone cheese
- ¼ cup of cocoa powder

Directions:

1. Take a big bowl; combine the melted chocolate with the ghee, eggs, swerve, cheese and cocoa. Whisk well, pour into a cake pan, introduce in the oven and cook at 375 degrees F for 25 minutes.
2. Cut into medium brownies and serve.

Nutrition: Calories 120 kcal Fat: 8 g Carbs: 3 g Protein: 3 g

100. Chocolate Cake with Blueberry

Preparation time: 10 minutes

Cooking time: 40 minutes

Servings: 8

Ingredients:

- 2 eggs, stripped into whites and yolks
- 25 g of cocoa powder
- 50 g of almond flour
- 20 g of flax flour
- 1 tsp. of sweetener (or to taste)
- 150 g of sour cream
- 50 g of vegetable oil
- 2 tsp. of baking powder
- Vanilla or vanilla extract to taste

Directions:

1. Turn on the oven to 180 degrees.
2. Beat the squirrel to stable foam.
3. Beat yolks with sweetener.
4. Add sour cream and vegetable oil and mix.
5. Add all the dry ingredients and mix again, you can use a mixer.
6. Add proteins in two steps and mix them gently into the dough.
7. Use the form 16 cm in diameter.
8. Put in the oven for 25 minutes.
9. Cut the cake into two. You can soak them with a mixture of 1 tbsp. of water and 1 tsp. of Liquor.
10. For the cream, beat all ingredients with a mixer.
11. Spread the cake and put the cake in the fridge to soak over the night.

Nutrition: Calories: 295.50 kcal Fat: 27.65 g Carbs: 7, 94 g Protein: 7.25 g

101. Chocolate Mousse

Preparation time: 5 minutes

Cooking time: 5 minutes

Servings: 4

Ingredients:

- 1 tbsp. of cocoa powder
- 2 oz. of cream cheese
- 2 oz. of butter
- 3 oz. of heavy whipping cream
- Stevia to taste

Directions:

1. Melt the butter a bit and mix with the sweetener. Stir until blended.
2. Add the cream cheese and cocoa powder and blend until smooth.
3. Carefully whip heavy cream and gradually add to the mixture.
4. Refrigerate it for 30 minutes.

Nutrition: Calories: 227 kcal Fat: 24 g Carbs: 3 g Protein: 4 g

102. Coconut Raspberry Cake

Preparation time: 1 hour and 10 minutes

Cooking time: 10 Minutes.

Servings: 6

Ingredients:

For the biscuit:

- 2 cups almond flour
- 1 egg
- 1 tablespoon of ghee, melted
- ½ teaspoon of baking soda

For the coconut layer:

- 1 cup of coconut milk
- ¼ cup of coconut oil, melted
- 3 cups coconut, shredded
- 1/3 cup of stevia
- 5 grams of food gelatin

For the raspberry layer:

- 1 cup of raspberries
- 1 teaspoon of stevia
- 3 tablespoons of chia seeds
- 5 grams of food gelatin

Directions:

1. In a bowl, combine the almond flour with the eggs, ghee and baking soda; stir well. Press on the bottom of the spring form

pan, and introduce in the oven at 350 degrees F for 15 minutes. Leave aside to cool down.

2. Meanwhile, in a pan, combine the raspberries with 1-teaspoon stevia, chia seeds, and gelatin; stir, and cook for 5 minutes. Take off the heat, cool down and spread over the biscuit layer.

3. In another small pan, combine the coconut milk with the coconut, oil, gelatin, 1/3 cup stevia; stir for 1-2 minutes. Take off the heat, cool down and spread over the coconut milk.

4. Cool the cake in the fridge for 1 hour, slice and serve.

Nutrition: Calories: 241 kcal Fat: 12 g Fiber: 4 g Carbs: 5 g Protein: 5 g

103.   Chickpea Choco Slices

Preparation time: 10 minutes

Cooking time: 50 minutes

Servings: 12 slices, 2 per serving

Ingredients:

- 400g can chickpeas,
- Rinsed, drained 250g almond butter
- 70ml maple syrup
- 15ml vanilla paste
- 1 pinch salt
- 2g baking powder
- 2g baking soda
- 40g vegan chocolate chips

Directions:

1. Preheat oven to 180C/350F.
2. Grease large baking pan with coconut oil.
3. Combine chickpeas, almond butter, maple syrup, vanilla, salt, baking powder, and baking soda in a food blender.
4. Blend until smooth. Stir in half the chocolate chips-
5. Spread the batter into the prepared baking pan.
6. Sprinkle with reserved chocolate chips.
7. Bake for 45-50 minutes or until an inserted toothpick comes out neat.
8. Appease on a wire rack for twenty minutes. slice and serve.

Nutrition: Calories 426 Total Fat 27.2g Total Carbohydrate 39.2g Dietary Fiber 4.9g Total Sugars 15.7g Protein 10g

104.　Sweet Green Cookies

Preparation time: 10 minutes

Cooking time: 30 minutes

Servings: 12 cookies, 3 per serving

Ingredients:

- 165g green peas
- 80g chopped Medjool dates
- 60g silken tofu, mashed
- 100g almond flour
- 1 teaspoon baking powder
- 12 almonds

Directions:

1. Preheat oven to 180C/350F.
2. Combine peas and dates in a food processor.
3. Process until the thick paste is formed.
4. Transfer the pea mixture into a bowl. Stir in tofu, almond flour, and baking powder.
5. Shape the mixture into 12 balls.
6. Arrange balls onto baking sheet, lined with parchment paper. Flatten each ball with oiled palm.
7. Insert an almond into each cookie. Bake the cookies for twenty-five to thirty minutes or until gently golden.
8. Cool on a wire rack before serving.

Nutrition: Calories 221 Total Fat 10.3g Total Carbohydrate 26.2g Dietary Fiber 6g Total Sugars 15.1g Protein 8.2g

105. Chickpea Cookie Dough

Preparation time: 10 minutes

Cooking time: 0 minutes

Servings: 4

Ingredients:

- 400g can chickpeas, rinsed, drained
- 130g smooth peanut butter
- 10ml vanilla extract
- ½ teaspoon cinnamon
- 10g chia seeds
- 40g quality dark Vegan chocolate chips

Direction:

1. Drain chickpeas in a colander.
2. Remove the skin from the chickpeas.
3. Place chickpeas, peanut butter, vanilla, cinnamon, and chia in a food blender.
4. Blend until smooth.
5. Stir in chocolate chips and divide among four serving bowls.
6. Serve.

Nutrition: Calories 376 Total Fat 20.9g Total Carbohydrate 37.2g Dietary Fiber 7.3g Total Sugars 3.3g Protein 14.2g

106.   Banana Bars

Preparation time: 10 minutes

Cooking time: 30 minutes

Servings: 8

Ingredients:

- 130g smooth peanut butter
- 60ml maple syrup
- 1 banana, mashed
- 45ml water
- 15g ground flax seeds
- 95g cooked quinoa
- 25g chia seeds
- 5ml vanilla
- 90g quick cooking oats
- 55g whole-wheat flour
- 5g baking powder
- 5g cinnamon
- 1 pinch salt
- Topping:
- 5ml melted coconut oil
- 30g vegan chocolate, chopped

Directions:

1. Preheat oven to 180C/350F.
2. Line 16cm baking dish with parchment paper.

3. Put together water and flax seeds in a small bowl. Place aside 10 minutes.

4. In a separate bowl, combine peanut butter, maple syrup, and banana. Fold in the flax seeds mixture.

5. Once you have a smooth mixture, stir in quinoa, chia seeds, vanilla extract, oat, whole-wheat flour, baking powder, cinnamon, and salt.

6. Pour the batter into prepared baking dish. Cut into 8 bars.

7. Bake the bars for 30 minutes.

8. In the meantime, make the topping; combine chocolate and coconut oil in a heatproof bowl. Set over simmering water, until melted.

9. Remove the bars from the oven. Place on a wire rack for 15 minutes to cool.

10. Remove the bars from the baking dish, and drizzle with chocolate topping.

11. Serve.

Nutrition: Calories 278 Total Fat 11.9g Total Carbohydrate 35.5g Dietary Fiber 5.8g Total Sugars 10.8g Protein 9.4g

107. Protein Donuts

Preparation Time: 5 minutes
Cooking Time: 20 minutes
Servings: 10 donuts, 2 per serving

Ingredients:

- 85g coconut flour
- 110g vanilla flavored germinated brown rice protein powder
- 25g almond flour
- 50g maple sugar
- 30ml melted coconut oil
- 8g baking powder
- 115ml soy milk
- ½ teaspoon apple cider vinegar
- ½ teaspoon vanilla paste
- ½ teaspoon cinnamon
- 30ml organic applesauce
- Additional:
- 30g powdered coconut sugar
- 10g cinnamon

Directions:

1. Add all the dried ingredients in a large cup.
2. In a separate bowl, whisk the milk with applesauce, coconut oil, and cider vinegar.
3. Fold the wet ingredients into dry and stir until blended thoroughly.
4. Heat oven to 180C/350F and grease 10-hole donut pan.
5. Spoon the prepared batter into greased donut pan.
6. Bake the donuts for 15-20 minutes.
7. Sprinkle with coconut sugar and cinnamon while the donuts are still warm,
8. Serve warm.

Nutrition: Calories 270 Total Fat 9.3g Total Carbohydrate 28.4g Dietary Fiber 10.2g Total Sugars 10.1g Protein 20.5g

108. Lentil Balls

Preparation time: 10 minutes

Cooking time: 0 minutes

Servings: 16 balls, 2 per serving

Ingredients:

- 150g cooked green lentils
- 10ml coconut oil
- 5g coconut sugar
- 180g quick cooking oats
- 40g unsweetened coconut, shredded
- 40g raw pumpkin seeds
- 110g peanut butter
- 40ml maple syrup

Directions:

1. Add all ingredients in a large bowl, as listed.
2. Shape the mixture into 16 balls.
3. Arrange the balls onto a plate, lined with parchment paper.
4. Refrigerate 30 minutes.
5. Serve.

Nutrition: Calories 305 Total Fat 13.7g 1 Total Carbohydrate 35.4g Dietary Fiber 9.5g Total Sugars 6.3g Protein 12.6g

109. Homemade granola

Preparation time: 10 minutes

Cooking time: 24 minutes

Servings: 8

Ingredients:

- 270g rolled oats
- 100g coconut flakes
- 40g pumpkin seeds
- 80g hemp seeds
- 30ml coconut oil
- 70ml maple syrup
- 50g Goji berries

Direction:

1. Add all ingredients on a large baking sheet.
2. Preheat oven to 180C°/350F.
3. Bake the granola for 12 minutes. Remove from the oven and stir.
4. Bake an additional 12 minutes.
5. Serve at room temperature.

Nutrition: Calories 344 Total Fat 17.4g Total Carbohydrate 39.7g Dietary Fiber 5.8g Total Sugars 12.9g Protein 9.9g

110. Cookie Almond Balls

Preparation time: 15 minutes

Cooking time: 0 minutes

Servings: 16 balls, 2 per serving

Ingredients:

- 100g almond meal
- 60g vanilla flavored rice protein powder
- 80g almond butter or any nut butter
- 10 drops Stevia
- 15ml coconut oil
- 15g coconut cream
- 40g vegan chocolate chips

Directions:

1. Combine almond meal and protein powder in a large bowl.
2. Fold in almond butter, Stevia, coconut oil, and coconut cream.
3. If the mixture is too crumbly, add some water. Fold in chopped chocolate and stir until combined.
4. Shape the mixture into 16 balls.
5. You can additional roll the balls into almond flour.
6. Serve.

Nutrition: Calories 132 Total Fat 8.4g Total Carbohydrate 6.7g Dietary Fiber 2.2g Total Sugars 3.1g Protein 8.1g

111.   Spiced Dutch Cookies

Preparation time: 20 minutes

Cooking time: 8 minutes

Servings: 6

Ingredients:

- 180g almond flour
- 55ml coconut oil, melted
- 60g rice protein powder, vanilla flavor
- 1 banana, mashed 40g Chia seeds
- Spice mix: 15g allspice
- 1 pinch white pepper
- 1 pinch ground coriander seeds
- 1 pinch ground mace

Directions:

1. Preheat oven to 190C/375F.
2. Soak chia seeds in ½ cup water. Place aside 10 minutes.
3. Mash banana in a large bowl.
4. Fold in almond flour, coconut oil, protein powder, and spice mix.
5. Add soaked chia seeds and stir to combine.
6. Stir until the dough is combined and soft. If needed add 1-2 tablespoons water.
7. Roll the dough to 1cm thick. Cut out cookies.
8. Arrange the cookies onto baking sheet, lined with parchment paper.
9. Bake 7-8 minutes.
10. Serve at room temperature.

Nutrition: Calories 278 Total Fat 20g Total Carbohydrate 13.1g Dietary Fiber 5.9g Total Sugars 2.4g Protein 13.1g

Two-Week Meal Plan

Week 1

Shopping List

1. Vegetables

Fresh produce can spoil quickly, so try to avoid over-purchasing whenever possible. If needed, fresh herbs can be swapped for the dried version. Plan to use leftover ingredients as an option for snacks throughout the week or to add more veggies to your entrées and side dishes.

- Alfalfa sprouts (1 container)
- Asparagus (1 small bunch)
- Avocados (2)
- Bell peppers, red (4)
- Carrots, shredded (1 bag)
- Cauliflower (1 head)
- Celery (1 bunch)
- Cucumbers (2)
- Dill, fresh (1 bunch)
- Garlic (1 bulb or jar)
- Green beans (1 pound)
- Kale (1 large bunch)
- Lettuce, romaine (1 head)
- Onion, yellow (1)
- Onions, red (2)

- Parsley, fresh (1 bunch)
- Potatoes, new (½ pound)
- Potatoes, yellow (2)
- Radishes (1 small bunch)
- Red cabbage, shredded (1 bag)
- Scallions (1 bunch)
- Spinach (1 large container)
- Tomato, Roma (1)
- Tomatoes, cherry (2 cups or 1 container)
- Zucchini (1 large)

2. Fruit

- Apples (2 or 3)
- Apricots, dried (½ cup)
- Lemons (2 or 3)
- Limes (1 or 2)
- Beans & Legumes
- Chickpeas, 1 (14.5-ounce) can
- Edamame, frozen, shelled (1 bag)
- Hummus (1 container)
- Split peas, green, dry (1¼ cups)

3. Whole Grains

- Bread, whole-wheat (1 loaf) or wraps (1 package)
- Freekeh, uncooked (1 cup)
- Oats, rolled, uncooked (1½ cups)

4. Seafood

- Cod, fillets, fresh or frozen, 4 (6-ounce) fillets
- Salmon, 2 (6-ounce) cans
- Salmon, smoked (4 ounces)
- Trout, smoked (8 ounces)
- Tuna, packed in water, 3 (5-ounce) cans

5. Nuts & Seeds

- Almonds, slivered (½ cup)
- Flaxseed, ground (¼ cup)
- Hemp hearts (1 bag)
- Pepitas (¼ cup)
- Pistachios, shelled (¼ cup)

6. Dairy & Eggs

- Cheese, goat or feta, crumbled (1 package)
- Cheese, pepper Jack, shredded (1 cup)
- Cheese, provolone or Gouda, sliced (1 package)
- Cream cheese, low-fat (1 block)
- Eggs, large (2 dozen)
- Yogurt, Greek, plain, low-fat (1 container)

7. Other Items

- Cereal, crisped rice (1 box)
- Chipotles in adobo sauce, 1 (7-ounce) can
- Coconut, unsweetened flakes (1 bag)
- Marinara sauce (1 jar)
- Salsa (1 jar)

- Tofu, firm, 1 (14-ounce) package

- Vegetable stock, low-sodium (1 quart)

- Wine, white (1 bottle)

	MONDAY	TUESDAY	WEDNESDAY
MORNING	Walnut Crunch Banana Bread	Whole-Wheat Blueberry Muffins	Walnut Crunch Banana Bread
MEAL 1	Lime Garlic Roasted Asparagus Easy Baked Tilapia	Parmesan and Wine Tilapia Eggplant Stacks	Scalloped Potatoes
MEAL 2	Eggplant Stacks Sanibel Southern Style	Celeriac Cauliflower Mash Sanibel Island Style Mussel	Beet Greens with Pine Nuts Goat Cheese
DESSERT	Coconut Raspberry Cake	Chocolate Mousse	Ice Cream with Avocado
DRINK	3L water	3L water	3L water

	THURSDAY	FRIDAY	SATURDAY	SUNDAY
MORNING	Plant-Powered Pancakes	Maple-Pecan Granola	Paradise Island Overnight Oatmeal	Pumpkin Pie Oatmeal
MEAL 1	Easy Baked Tilapia	Teriyaki Eggplant	Butter, Garlic, And Tomatoes Tilapia	Scalloped Potatoes
MEAL 2	Beet Greens with Pine Nuts Goat Cheese Halibut	Baked Cod & Green Beans French Mussels	Eggplant Stacks	Garlic Chive Cauliflower Mash
DESSERT	Ice Cream with Avocado	Delicious Brownies	Chocolate Cake with Blueberry	Chocolate Mousse
DRINK	**3L water**	**3L water**	**3L water**	**3L water**

Week 2

Shopping List

1. Vegetables

- Avocados (2)

- Beans, green (½ pound)

- Bell pepper, red (1)

- Cabbage, shredded (1 bag, or use leftovers from Week 1)

- Carrots, large (2)

- Carrots, shredded (1 bag, or use leftovers from Week 1)

- Celery (1 bunch)
- Cilantro, fresh (1 bunch)
- Corn, sweet kernels, frozen (1 bag) or 1 can
- Cucumbers (4)
- Garlic (1 head or jar)
- Kale, green (1 or 2 bunches)
- Leafy greens or spring mix (1 large container)
- Mint, fresh (1 bunch)
- Onion, yellow (1)
- Onions, red (2)
- Parsley, fresh (1 bunch)
- Potatoes, sweet (5 large)
- Scallions (1 bunch)
- Spinach, baby (1 bag)
- Tomatoes, cherry (1 container)
- Tomatoes, Roma (2)
- Tomatoes, sun-dried (1 bag)

2. **Fruit**

- Apples, Granny Smith
- Apricots, dried (¼ cup)
- Bananas (1 or 2)
- Blueberries, frozen (1 bag)
- Lemons (2 or 3)
- Limes (1 or 2)

- Peaches, frozen (1 bag)
- Raspberries (2 pints)

3. Beans & Legumes

- Beans, black, 1 (15.5-ounce) can
- Beans, cannellini or great northern, 1 (15.5-ounce) can
- Chickpeas, 2 (14.5-ounce) cans
- Edamame, frozen, shelled (1 bag, or use leftovers from Week 1)
- Hummus (1 container)
- Tempeh, 1 (8-ounce) package
- Tofu, firm, 2 (14-ounce) packages

4. Whole Grains

- Bread, whole-wheat (1 loaf)
- Bulgur, uncooked (½ cup)
- Oats, rolled, uncooked (3½ cups)
- Rice, brown, uncooked (3 cups)

5. Seafood

- Salmon, fresh or frozen, 4 (6-ounce) fillets
- Tuna, white, packed in water, 3 (5-ounce) cans

6. Nuts & Seeds

- Almonds, slivered (¾ cup)
- Pistachios, shelled (¼ cup)
- Sunflower seeds, roasted (½ cup)
- Tahini (1 jar)

Dairy & Eggs

- Cheese, Cheddar, sliced (1 package)

- Cheese, cottage, low-fat (1 container)

- Cheese, feta, crumbled (1 package, or use leftovers from Week 1)

- Eggs, large (1 dozen)

- Kefir, plain or vanilla (1 bottle)

- Yogurt, Greek, plain, low-fat (2 containers)

Other Items

- Chipotles in adobo sauce, 1 (7-ounce) can

- Coconut milk, 1 (13-ounce) can

- Tea, chai (1 box)

	MONDAY	TUESDAY	WEDNESDAY
MORNING	Chocolate and Peanut Butter Quinoa	A.M. Breakfast Scramble	Loaded Breakfast Burrito
MEAL 1	Spicy Garlic Tilapia	Potatoes and Mushrooms	Lime Garlic Roasted Asparagus
MEAL 2	Creamed Coconut Curry Spinach	Sautéed Carrot and Green Onions	Garlic Chive Cauliflower Mash
DESSERT	Coconut Raspberry Cake	Protein Donuts	Homemade Granola
DRINK	3L water	3L water	3L water

	THURSDAY	FRIDAY	SATURDAY	SUNDAY
MORNING	Whole-Wheat Blueberry Muffins	Walnut Crunch Banana Bread	Plant-Powered Pancakes	Maple-Pecan Granola
MEAL 1	Sautéed Carrot and Green Onions Spinach Soup with Dill and Basil	Hot and Sour Soup with Shrimp with lemongrass Potatoes and Mushrooms	Chickpeas and Rice	Lime Garlic Roasted Asparagus
MEAL 2	Beet Greens with Pine Nuts Goat Cheese	Eggplant Parmesan Whangarei Style	Celeria Cauliflower Mash Restaurant Style Halibut	Coconut Watercress Soup
DESSERT	Sweet Green Cookies	Chickpea Cookie Dough	Coconut Raspberry Cake	Spiced Dutch Cookies
DRINK	**3L water**	**3L water**	**3L water**	**3L water**

Conclusion

Now that you have reached the end of this cookbook, I am sure that you have learned a lot about the Pescatarian Diet, what foods to eat and what are the foods to avoid. This book has a lot to offer for you with the many healthy benefits of Pescatarian Diet.

Before we end this book, always remember the following key points that I want you to remember by heart.

A pescatarian is anyone who includes seafood and fish to the vegetarian diet. Different people, for several reasons, may decide to eliminate poultry and meat from their diet but still retain fish. Some vegetarians include fish to their food as they want to not only enjoy the benefits of a plant-based diet but also have a healthy heart. Some others may do this because it suits their taste. While the rest may stick to the pescatarian diet simply because of its impact on the environment.

In this book, we will look at what the pescatarian diet is all about, benefits of this diet, foods to eat and foods not to eat as well as a shopping list to help you succeed with the pescatarian diet. You will also enjoy delicious and easy to make dinner recipes as well as a 7-day meal plan for easy planning of your meals.

A pescatarian is someone that includes fish to their diet but avoids meat and other poultry. The term was coined in the early 1990s with a combination of two words, 'Pesce,' which means fish and 'vegetarian.' In summary, a pescatarian is anyone who follows the vegetarian diet, but also includes fish and other seafood to his or her diet. The diet is mainly made up of plant-based foods like legumes, healthy fats, nuts, whole grains, and produce with seafood being the major source of protein.

It may interest you to know that several pescatarians eat eggs and dairy too. In the same way that we have several versions of the vegetarian diet, we also have several versions of the pescatarian diet. One can eat a diet free of meat but packed with plenty of junk foods, processed starches, and fish sticks instead of a healthier diet made up of whole foods.

Dietary choices obviously play a big role in reducing the risk of adverse health outcomes.

Research has proven that plant-based diets have several advantages, including lowering the risk of obesity and chronic diseases like diabetes and heart disease. Research also shows that you can get these protective benefits from following the pescatarian diet.

One study proved that women who followed the pescatarian diet gained 2.5 fewer pounds than women who had meat included in their diet. Also, people who changed their diet to plant-based gained the least amount of weight. This means that reducing your consumption of meat and poultry may be beneficial to your health regardless of your current eating patterns.

Another study concluded that people on a pescatarian diet had reduced the risk of developing diabetes at 4.8 percent compared to omnivores at 7.6 percent.

Also, one study looked at people who were pescatarian or rarely ate meat, and it discovered that these people had a 22 percent lower risk of dying from heart diseases when compared to people who eat meat regularly.

People who are just beginning the pescatarian diet may find it difficult to design their meals for the next few weeks. This may cause some people to default to eating more of high carb meals, which is not the best way to maintain a healthy balanced diet. One of the great benefits of this diet is that you get to enjoy plenty of omega-3 fatty acids from fish, which will lower inflammation in the body.

Thanks again for reading this book. I hope it helped you a lot! Enjoy!

CPSIA information can be obtained
at www.ICGtesting.com
Printed in the USA
LVHW080754081220
672143LV00036B/335

9 781914 017599